PAIN MANAGEMENT - RESEARCH AND TECHNOLOGY

PAIN MANAGEMENT

RECENT INTERNATIONAL RESEARCH

Pain Management - Research and Technology

Additional books and e-books in this series can be found on Nova's website under the Series tab.

PAIN MANAGEMENT - RESEARCH AND TECHNOLOGY

PAIN MANAGEMENT

RECENT INTERNATIONAL RESEARCH

JOAV MERRICK

AND

MOHAMMED MORAD

EDITORS

nova

Medicine & Health

https://doi.org/10.52305/YMJQ2632

Library of Congress Cataloging-in-Publication Data

ISBN: 978-1-68507-493-7

Published by Nova Science Publishers, Inc. † New York

Contents

INTRODUCTION

In: Pain Management
Editors: J Merrick and M Morad
ISBN: 978-1-68507-493-7

Chapter 1

PAIN AND PAIN MANAGEMENT

Joav Merrick[1-4,*], MD, MMedSci, DMSc and Mohammed Morad[2,5,6], MD, FRCP

[1]Department of Pediatrics, Mt Scopus Campus, Hadassah Hebrew University Medical Center, Jerusalem, Israel
[2]National Institute of Child Health and Human Development, Jerusalem, Israel
[3]Kentucky Children's Hospital, University of Kentucky, Lexington, Kentucky, United States of America
[4]Center for Healthy Development, School of Public Health, Georgia State University, Atlanta, United States of America
[5]Clalit Health Services
[6]Department of Family Medicine, Division of Community Health, Faculty of Health Sciences, Ben Gurion University of the Negev, Beer Sheva, Israel

* ***Correspondence:*** Professor Joav Merrick, MD, MMedSci, DMSc, Director, National Institute of Child Health and Human Development, Jerusalem, Israel.
Email: jmerrick@zahav.net.il.

Abstract

Before neurons and their role in pain there have been many explanations to account for pain. Hippocrates (370-460 BCE) believed that it was due to an imbalance in vital fluids and in the 11th century Avicenna (980-1037) theorized that there were a number of feeling senses including touch, pain and titillation. Today we talk about four types of pain: 1) Nociceptive pain: Typically the result of tissue injury, 2) Inflammatory pain: An abnormal inflammation caused by an inappropriate response by the body's immune system, 3) Neuropathic pain: Pain caused by nerve irritation and 4) Functional pain: Pain without obvious origin, but can cause pain. About 20% of adults had chronic pain and 7% of adults had chronic pain that frequently limit life or work activities, which increase with age. In this book we have gathered recent international research on pain and pain management from internationally renowned researchers from around the world, which we hope will be of interest to the reader.

Introduction

The International Association for the Study of Pain defines pain as "an unpleasant sensory and emotional experience associated with, or resembling that associated with, actual or potential tissue damage" (1).

Before neurons and their role in pain there have been many explanations to account for pain. Hippocrates (370-460 BCE) believed that it was due to an imbalance in vital fluids and in the 11th century Avicenna (980-1037) theorized that there were a number of feeling senses including touch, pain and titillation (1).

Around 1644 René Descartes (1596-1650) thought that pain was a disturbance that passed down along nerve fibers until the disturbance reached the brain (1). In the 18th and 19th centuries came the intensive theory, which conceived of pain not as a unique sensory modality, but an emotional state produced by stronger than normal stimuli such as intense light, pressure or temperature (1). By the mid-1890s, specificity was backed mostly by physiologists and physicians, and the intensive theory was mostly backed by psychologists (1).

Today we talk about four types of pain: 1) Nociceptive pain: Typically the result of tissue injury. Common types of nociceptive pain are arthritis pain, mechanical back pain or post-surgical pain, 2) Inflammatory pain: An abnormal inflammation caused by an inappropriate response by the body's immune system. Conditions in this category include gout and rheumatoid arthritis, 3) Neuropathic pain: Pain caused by nerve irritation. This includes conditions such as neuropathy, radicular pain and trigeminal neuralgia and 4) Functional pain: Pain without obvious origin, but can cause pain. Examples of such conditions are fibromyalgia or irritable bowel syndrome.

SURVEY DATA

Data from the National Center for Health Statistics and the National Health Interview Survey (2) showed that in the United States in 2019:

- 20.4% of adults had chronic pain and 7.4% of adults had chronic pain that frequently limited life or work activities (referred to as high impact chronic pain) in the past three months.
- Chronic pain and high-impact chronic pain both increased with age and were highest among adults aged 65 years and older.
- Non-Hispanic white adults (23.6%) were more likely to have chronic pain compared with non-Hispanic black (19.3%), Hispanic (13.0%), and non-Hispanic Asian (6.8%) adults.
- The percentage of adults with chronic pain and high-impact chronic pain increased as place of residence became more rural.

Chronic pain and chronic pain that frequently limits life or work activities are among the most common reasons adults seek medical care and are associated with decreased quality of life, opioid dependence and poor mental health (2). Women were more likely to have chronic pain (21.7%) and high-impact chronic pain (8.5%) compared with men (19.0% and 6.3%, respectively) (2).

In this book

In this book we have gathered recent international research on pain and pain management from internationally renowned researchers from around the world, which we hope will be of interest to the reader.

References

[1] Wikipedia. Pain. URL: https://en.wikipedia.org/wiki/Pain.

[2] Zelaya CE, Dahlhamer JM, Lucas JW, Connor EM. Chronic pain and high-impact chronic pain among US adults, 2019. NCHS Data Brief 390, Nov 2020.

SECTION ONE: PAIN MANAGEMENT

In: Pain Management
Editors: J Merrick and M Morad
ISBN: 978-1-68507-493-7

Chapter 2

THE ASSOCIATIONS OF PAIN CATASTROPHIZING AND POST-OPERATIVE OUTCOMES IN DOMAINS OF PAIN, QUALITY OF LIFE AND FUNCTION IN JOINT REPLACEMENT SURGERY

Lorelle Dismore**, MBPsS, Anna van Wersch, PhD, Rebecca Critchley, MRCS, Aradhyula An Murty, FRCS and Katherine Swainston, PhD

Department of Research and Development,
Northumbria Healthcare NHS Foundation Trust,
North Tyneside General Hospital, Rake Lane, North Shields,
Tyne and Wear and School of Social Sciences,
Humanities and Law, Teesside University, Campus Heart,
Southfield Road, Middlesbrough, England

* ***Correspondence:*** Lorelle Dismore, MBPsS, Health Psychologist, Department of Research and Development, Northumbria Healthcare NHS Foundation Trust, North Tyneside General Hospital, Rake Lane, North Shields, Tyne and Wear, NE29 8NH, United Kingdom, 0191 293 4087 Email: Lorelle.dismore@northumbria-healthcare.nhs.uk.

ABSTRACT

The National Institute for Health and Care Excellence (NICE) guidelines aim to identify the best approach for recovery and rehabilitation to enable clinicians to treat patients more effectively and efficiently. Identification of the pre-surgical modifiable psychosocial risk factors that impact on post-operative recovery offers an opportunity to develop effective and appropriate interventions to facilitate patient's recovery, which in turn will improve outcomes. A psychological construct termed pain catastrophizing has been identified as a unique predictor of chronic post-surgical pain. The clinical importance of pain catastrophizing in moderating surgical outcomes is well documented in musculoskeletal disorders and is considered one of the key predictors of post-operative pain intensity, delayed recovery, poorer quality of life and perceived disability. Objective: To identify whether pain catastrophizing affects post-surgical outcomes following joint replacement surgery in relation to pain, function and quality of life. Study group: joint replacement surgery. Methods: Systematic review identifying eight studies assessing catastrophizing and post-operative outcomes in domains of pain, quality of life and/or function. Results: The analysis of the results are limited to a qualitative synthesis of the eligible studies. Pain catastrophizing was associated with all domains; patients with high pain catastrophizing symptoms were more symptomatic post-surgery, experienced more pain and rated themselves as dissatisfied; dissatisfied patients experienced lower quality of life. Pain catastrophizing is a useful prognostic indicator for identifying individuals at-risk for poorer post-operative outcomes. Conclusions: A multidisciplinary approach with an appropriate intervention to reduce catastrophizing symptoms preoperatively may optimise post-operative outcomes following joint replacement.

INTRODUCTION

In 2017/2018 more joint replacements than previous years were carried out, with over 252,000 cases submitted to the National Joint Registry, 92 per cent of primary joint replacements procedures were for osteoarthritis, and more of them in women. The number of procedures performed has significantly increased by almost 10,000 joint replacement operations from previous periods (1). Given the rapid increase in joint replacements the National Institute for Health and Care Excellence (NICE) are developing clinical guidelines on hip, knee and shoulder joint replacement. The guidelines will identify the best approach for recovery and rehabilitation to enable clinicians to treat patients more effectively and efficiently (2). In patients undergoing knee replacement surgery, up to 30% have been identified as experiencing a suboptimal outcome or rate themselves as dissatisfied (3), often influenced by psychological factors (4). To optimise post-operative outcomes, identification of modifiable psychosocial risk factors that impact on patient's recovery offers opportunities to develop effective and appropriate interventions. One psychological construct termed pain catastrophizing (PC) has consistently been identified as influencing surgical outcomes (5).

Catastrophizing is a coping style defined as "an exaggerated negative mental set brought to bear during actual or anticipated painful experience" (6). It is a cognitive emotional process, unrelated to spinal nociception, which can result in heightened emotional stress. Catastrophizing is measured using the pain catastrophizing scale (PCS), it is a multidimensional construct comprising of three elements of rumination "I can't seem to keep it out of my mind and magnification "I keep thinking of other painful events," which refer to experiencing painful stimuli as extremely threatening and helplessness "I feel I can't go on" which refers to the inability to cope with painful stimuli. Respondents can score a possible score of zero to fifty-two, with higher scores indicating higher catastrophizing symptoms.

A growing amount of literature demonstrates the associations of PC with various health outcomes, including delayed recovery in patients with low back pain, pain-related disability, poorer reported pain control, and increased pain severity, reduced quality of life (QoL) and longer hospital stay (7-13). Patients who catastrophize about their symptoms may prompt healthcare professionals to pursue more intensive and invasive approaches to pain assessment and treatment (6), and there are associated health care costs resulting from specialist consultation and use of pain medication for musculoskeletal pain (14).

Catastrophizing has been well documented as moderating surgical outcomes (15). Predicting acute post-operative pain following lumbar fusion surgery, hysterectomy, abdominal surgery, cardiac surgery, and breast cancer surgery (12, 16-19). Patients who catastrophize are more likely to report taking opioid pain medications two months post-surgery regardless of injury severity, fracture site or treating surgeon (20), and greater analgesic use following breast cancer surgery (12). Studies of longer follow ups in various surgical procedures have demonstrated that individuals with high PC symptoms experience increased pain severity, greater incidence of chronic post-surgical pain (CPSP) (8), and poorer QoL and function (21, 22).

There is variability in the cut-off points used to identify problematic catastrophizing in surgical models. For example, scores of above 13 have been demonstrated as predictive of acute post-operative pain following cruciate ligament repair (23). Scores of 16 or higher were predictive of CPSP following knee arthroplasty (24). Other surgical studies have used scores of 20 (3), 30 and above (25) or have examined PC as a continuous variable without guidance for cut-scores (26). Identifying and reducing PC levels in the pre-operative period may help to optimise post-operative outcomes in surgical patients and enhance improvements in changes in disability and pain (5, 27). Due to the variability of cut-scores across different surgical procedures, there are potential problems arising in distinguishing high versus low catastrophizing and when to intervene with appropriate interventions. Additionally, there are differences in studies demonstrating significant differences as opposed to meaningful clinically important differences (MCID). MCID are patient derived scores that reflect changes in a clinical intervention that are meaningful for the patient (28). On average, a reduction of two points or 30% represent MCID when measuring pain (29).

Majority of the surgical studies conducted are in hip and knee arthroplasty. It is well documented that there is an association with PC and post-operative pain (21). In this review, we report the associations with PC and post-operative outcomes following joint replacement surgery in relation to pain, and in addition QoL and/or function.

OUR STUDY

A systematic search strategy was employed using databases; PsychInfo, Embase, Medline, PubMed and CINAHL (range date until April 2020). The search terms were "catastrophize*" OR "catastrophizing" AND "pain", AND "surgery" OR "post-surgical" OR "chronic" AND "outcome*" OR "evaluation" (appendix). Grey literature was sought using Google Scholar and all reference lists of the included articles were checked to ensure literature saturation.

Example of search strategy

Draft PsycINFO search

- 1. ("pain").ti,ab
- 2. (catastrophize*).ti,ab
- 3. (catastrophizing).ti,ab
- 4. (2 OR 3)
- 5. (1 AND 4)
- 6. (surgery).ti,ab
- 7. ("post surgery").ti,ab
- 8. (chronic).ti,ab
- 9. (6 OR 7 OR 8)
- 10. (outcome*).ti,ab
- 11. (evaluation).ti,ab
- 12. (10 OR 11)
- 13. (9 AND 12)
- 14. (5 AND 13)

Study inclusion and exclusion criteria

Inclusion criteria were as follows; participants 18 years or older, undergoing joint replacement surgery, published in the English language, and had primarily measured PC and patient reported outcome measures (PROMs). PROMs are indicators for measuring post-operative outcomes and usually take into account pain, function, range of motion, stability, mobility and/or QoL. PROMs had to measure at least one out of three outcomes; pain, function and/or health related QoL. Observational cohort studies were included and had to incorporate a comparison group to enable identification of problematic outcomes in those patients reaching suboptimal recovery versus optimal recovery. Follow-up data must have been collected for at least three months post-surgery to allow for a sufficient timeframe to observe an effect. It has been suggested that patients have a rapid recovery the first three to four months following total hip arthroplasty, but improvements continue at a slower rate for up to a year (30). Therefore, articles were excluded that assessed short-term effects (<3 months). Other exclusions included: reviews, trial protocol description, conference abstracts, book chapters, opinions or commentaries.

Figure 1 describes the study selection process (PRISM flow chart): 2,420 articles were identified through database searching, after removing 1,375 duplicates a total of 1,045 were reviewed by an independent author by title/abstract to ensure they met the inclusion criteria. For articles that met the inclusion criteria or where the reviewer lacked certainty full-text articles were requested. Fifty one articles were requested, forty three articles were excluded for reasons pertaining to; no comparison group, surgery for a condition of different aetiology (keyhole, spinal surgery and fractures), short-term follow up, participants received therapy, the primary aim was the length of hospital stay and discharge and an assessment of the stability of PC, cohort comprising of surgery and conservative treatment, review and conference abstracts.

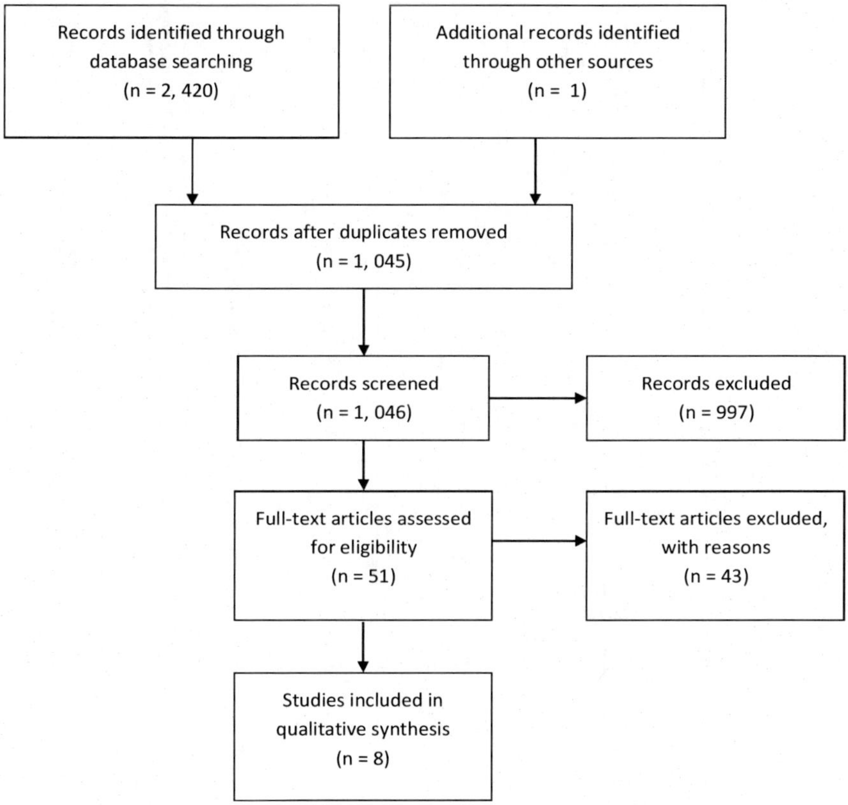

Figure 1. PRISM flow diagram.

Data extraction

A total of eight articles met the inclusion criteria. Methodological quality was assessed with the Critical Appraisal Skills Programme (CASP) Appraisal Checklist for a Cohort Study. The tool assesses three broad issues pertaining to the results of studies and checked by two authors.

While all eight included studies assessed pain as an outcome measure, four of these studies assessed and reported additional outcomes relating to function and QoL. These have been separated for the purposes of presentation of the review findings. Study characteristics and main findings are summarised in Table 1.

Table 1. Characteristics of all eligible publications

First Author, Year	N participants	Comparison Group	Surgical Procedure	Outcome measures & PCS cut off scores	Key Findings
Observational Cohort Studies					
Wright, (2017)	123 3 months; 119	High PC group to a low PC group	Primary TKA or THA	VAS PCS $\geq$ 30	Those who catastrophized scored 1.29 points higher than those who did not catastrophize at 3 months. However, there was no MCID between the groups in reported VAS.
Forsythe, (2008)	55 3 months; 43 12 months; 46 24 months; 48	Persistent pain group versus no pain	TKA	MPQ, PRI PCS; mean scores	Patients with persistent pain at 24 months had significantly higher preoperative PCS-rumination and total scores.
Dave, (2016)	267 12 months; 241	Regional body pain diagram groups	TKA	Pain diagram score, WOMAC PCS $\geq$ 20	PC scores contributed independently to suboptimal outcome.
Noiseux, (2014)	215 6 months; 193	Low, moderate and severe pain groups	TKA	NRS at rest and with ROM, PCS (mean scores)	PC significantly correlated with high levels of ongoing pain at 6 month's post-TKA.
Bierke, (2017)	138 6 months; 117 12 months; 100	High PC group to a low PC group	TKR	NRS, KOOS PCS >30	Pre-operative PC patients had poorer outcomes on pain and QoL and lower knee function before and after surgery.

First Author, Year	N participants	Comparison Group	Surgical Procedure	Outcome measures & PCS cut off scores	Key Findings
Van Onsem, (2016)	113 3 months; 113	Dissatisfied versus Satisfied patients	TKA	KOOS, OKS, EQ-5D, KSS PCS (mean scores)	Dissatisfied patients were more likely to ruminate and reported a tendency to perceive themselves as being unable to control pain symptoms.
Riddle, (2010)	157 6 months; 140	Patients who improved by ≥50% on changes in WOMAC pain and function scores	TKA	WOMAC PCS ≥ 16	High catastrophizing was associated with poorer post-operative pain outcomes.
Dhurve, (2017)	48	Dissatisfied versus Satisfied patients	TKA	OKS, VR-12 PCS; mean scores	Dissatisfied patients experienced higher postoperative PC scores and poorer functional improvements.

Abbreviations/Notes:

TKA, total knee arthroplasty; TKR, total knee replacement; THA, total hip arthroplasty; LSS, lumbar spine surgery; PCS, pain catastrophizing scale; VAS, visual analogue scale; MCID, minimally clinically important difference; NRS, numerical rating scale; KOOS, knee osteoarthritis outcome score; QoL, quality of life; PC, pain catastrophizing; OKS, oxford knee score; VR-12, Veterans Rand 12 item health survey; WOMAC, western Ontario and McMaster Universities osteoarthritis index; EQ-5D, health related quality of life; KSS, knee society score; ADL, activities of daily living; MPQ, the McGill questionnaire; PRI, pain rating index; ROM, range-of-motion.

FINDINGS

Of the four studies that assessed pain as an outcome measure, associations were observed with PC and post-operative pain. Two studies measured MCID in improvement in pain (3, 25).

Forsythe and colleagues aimed to determine if PC scores are predictive of long-term pain outcomes following total knee arthroplasty (TKA). Patients with persistent pain at 24-months post-TKA had significantly higher preoperative rumination scores and total PC scores and scores did not change from pre- to post-surgery (31). Similarly, Wright and colleagues conducted a study into the relationship between PC (scoring 30 or greater) and postoperative pain intensity with the inclusion of both knee and hip arthroplasty patients. A statistical significance in post-operative pain scores between catastrophizers and non-catastrophizers was observed. Individuals with high catastrophizing symptoms scored 1.29 points higher than those who did not catastrophize (25). However, when using MCID criteria of two there was no difference between both groups in reported pain scores 3-months post-surgery. Whereas, Dave and colleagues identified problematic outcomes in patients failing to achieve the estimated MCID assessed by reductions in WOMAC pain scores and found 12% of 241 patients reached suboptimal recovery 12-months following TKA. PC scores contributed independently to suboptimal outcome (3). Noiseux and colleagues examined pain during movement and found PC scores significantly correlated with high levels of on-going pain at 6-month's post-TKA. Sixteen per cent of 193 patients had moderate to severe pain with a range-of-motion test. Patients with moderate to severe pain post-TKA experienced greater PC symptoms pre-operatively (32). There is evidence for an association between PC and post-operative pain, however of the two studies using MCID the evidence is contradictory and further research is warranted.

Pain, function and quality of life

Of the four studies that included pain and additional outcomes for function and QoL, two showed an association with PC (33, 34), one study showed an association with the rumination subscale of the PCS (35) and one study showed an association with PC and pain but not function (36).

Of the three studies showing associations with all domains, Bierke and Petersen evaluated PC in relation to post-operative outcomes following total knee replacement (TKR). Patients scoring 30 or above had poorer outcomes compared to patients not experiencing catastrophizing symptoms and were more dissatisfied (33). Dhurve and colleagues were also interested in dissatisfaction following TKR and found dissatisfied patients experienced higher postoperative PC scores and poorer functional improvements. Reasons and outcomes associated with dissatisfaction included on-going pain, followed by stiffness and expectations not met (34). Van Onsem et al., classified predictors of patient satisfaction and found 12% of 113 patients were dissatisfied 3-months following TKA. Dissatisfied patients were more likely to ruminate, experienced lower QoL, were more symptomatic and perceived themselves as being unable to control pain symptoms (35). Riddle and colleagues were interested in changes in improvements in WOMAC pain and function scores by 50% or greater and found patients with high PC scores of 16 or greater had poorer post-operative pain outcomes but not function 6-months post-TKA (36). Overall, there is a limited amount of evidence examining the associations between PC, and pain, QoL and/or function.

CONCLUSION AND DISCUSSION

There is growing evidence in the literature that shows how PC moderates surgical outcomes in both the acute and chronic pain population. Much of the previous literature has focused on PC and post-operative pain severity in hip and knee arthroplasty. This review found not only the associations of PC and post-operative pain, but in addition issues pertaining to function and QoL in patients receiving surgery for knee or hip replacement.

The main findings amongst the studies demonstrated that dissatisfied patients who did not achieve optimal outcome experienced high catastrophizing symptoms and of the one study that assessed the subscales of the PCS, scored highly on the rumination subscale. Patients with high catastrophizing symptoms tend to perceive themselves as being unable to control pain symptoms and report being more symptomatic with less improvement in activities of daily living, mobility and usual activities. Pre-operative PC predicted post-operative pain, poorer functional improvements, and disability, with subsequent negative effects on patients QoL.

Catastrophizing is clinically important however, six of the studies did not measure MCID (31-36), in order to indicate whether changes in patients' PROMs can result in changes in their care and treatment. Of the three studies measuring MCID, Dave and colleagues indicated 12% of 241 patients reached suboptimal recovery 12-months following TKA (PC scores of higher than 20 or above). Whereas, Wright and colleagues found a significant difference in pain scores following total joint arthroplasty in those with high PC scores (scoring 30 or above) versus those with lower scores, but pain scores were not of clinical importance (25). The authors suggest PC scores are a poor predictor for post-operative pain. However, the differences in findings may be attributed to the sample of a mixed cohort of patients receiving hip or knee replacement. Riddle et al., found patients with high PC scores (16 or greater) had poorer post-operative pain, but not function 6-months following TKA. This was the only study measuring MCID that included additional outcome measures other than pain, with the inclusion of a PC cut-off score of 16 to identify problematic outcomes. Consistent with the previous literature, this review found that there was variability in PC measurements of the optimal cut-off scores in surgical models to identify problematic outcomes. The differences in findings may therefore be attributed to the variability in cut-scores and it becomes less clear as to who would be classified as demonstrating high catastrophizing symptoms. Some patients included in some studies would not be included in others, or would be classified using a different score. The lowest cut-off score of 16 demonstrated problematic outcomes and may be a useful starting point when considering who would benefit from behavioural interventions to optimise surgical outcomes.

There are strengths and limitations to the studies and the variation in findings may be attributed to the differences in study methodologies. For example, the inconsistencies in outcome measures, heterogeneous samples, and only one study included hip replacement patients. Additionally, literature highlights that patients with lower preoperative radiographic osteoarthritis undergoing total joint arthroplasty are more likely to experience high pain post-surgery (37). Arthritis grading was not accounted for in all of the included studies as a possible confounding variable, therefore limiting the validity of the findings (3, 25, 31, 36).

Limitations of this review include; the analysis of the results were limited to a qualitative synthesis of the eligible studies, and a meta-analysis was not performed due to the clinical and methodological heterogeneity. The inclusion criteria of the studies requiring a comparison group in order to detect changes in outcomes. This was due to the inconsistencies across the studies. For example, comparison groups related to the outcome (pain versus no pain group) or the predictor variable (high versus low PC). This therefore reduced the amount of studies included but previous reviews have already highlighted the associations between PC and post-operative pain. Accordingly, this review aimed to explore the associated factors pertaining to why some patients reach optimal versus suboptimal outcome with the inclusion of QoL and functional outcome measures. Future research could focus on demonstrating the key differences and associated factors between high and low catastrophizing, but with the use of optimal scores that constitute high symptoms of catastrophizing.

In this review, there is evidence to support PC as a stable (trait) and dynamic (state) variable. For example, where PC scores did not change from pre- to post-surgery as opposed to pain scores having decreased PC is supported as remaining stable over time (trait). However, studies that did not collect pre-operative PC scores, cannot determine if PC symptoms develop due to unfavourable outcomes or reflect a pre-operative state (dynamic). Nevertheless, a state variable is potentially modifiable, supporting the use of behavioural interventions to optimise post-operative outcomes. Interventional studies would help determine the most appropriate timing (pre- or post-surgery).

The majority of the included studies were recently published, highlighting the current approach to understanding modifiable psychosocial factors impacting post-operative outcomes. Recognition is given towards the implications of PC as a maladaptive coping style. Seven studies recommend PC as a useful prognostic indicator to identify individuals at risk of poorer post-operative outcomes. However, results should be treated with caution when considering hip replacement patients and more research is needed within this population with the inclusion of QoL and functional outcome measures. Van Onsem and colleagues have developed a prediction tool to assist in patient selection with the inclusion of rumination (35). The PCS is also a better predictor compared to surgeon's being able to identify low or high levels of catastrophizing, in orthopaedic patients after routine clinical consultation (38).

In the UK, more women have undergone joint replacement than men (1) and experience lower satisfaction, often associated with pain and stiffness in a TKA population (39). The mean age at implantation in women and men is 68 years and 68.9 years, respectively. However, patients requiring joint replacement surgery are getting younger and are more likely to undergo revision (1). In helping patients reach optimal recovery a multidisciplinary approach is needed to treat all modifiable components of the patient's overall health, with a shift from a medical model of surgery to a biopsychosocial model. Interviewing patients to understand why they may experience high catastrophizing symptoms and their associated psychosocial factors impacting on their recovery would be invaluable and may help when designing behavioural interventions. As well as understanding the views of orthopaedic practitioners providing care, such as their thoughts towards PC and how to improve surgical practice.

We identified eight studies that provide support for PC moderating post-operative outcomes in pain function and/or QoL, largely in TKA populations. An identification of at-risk patients using an optimal PCS cut-score would aid patient selection for behavioural interventions. The lowest PC score of 16 demonstrated as problematic and may be a useful starting score. Catastrophizing is clinically relevant and modifiable and patients should be treated with a multidisciplinary approach to enhance and optimise their post-operative outcomes.

ACKNOWLEDGMENTS

We would like to thank Mr Keith Gray for his assistance and guidance in this review and acknowledge BOFAS.

REFERENCES

[1] Healthcare Quality Improvement Partnership. The National Joint Registry for England, Wales, Northern Ireland and the Isle of Man. London: NJR 15th Annual Report, 2018.

[2] National Institute for Health and Care Excellence online. NICE guideline: Joint replacement (primary): hip, knee and shoulder final scope. URL: hwww.nice.org.uk/guidance/gid-ng10084/documents/final-scope-2.

[3] Dave AJ, Selzer F, Losina E, Usiskin I, Collins JE, Lee YC, et al. The association of pre-operative body pain diagram scores with pain outcomes following total knee arthroplasty. Osteoarthritis Cartilage 2017;25(5):667-75.

[4] Vissers MM, Bussmann JB, Verhaar JA, Busschbach JJ, Bierma-Zeinstra SM, Reijman M. Psychological factors affecting the outcome of total hip and knee arthroplasty: a systematic review. Semin Arthritis Rheum 2012;41(4):576-88.

[5] Khan RS, Ahmed K, Blakeway E, Skapinakis P, Nihoyannopoulos L, Macleod K, et al. Catastrophizing: A predictive factor for postoperative pain. Am J Surgery 2011;201(1):122-31.

[6] Sullivan MJL. The Pain Catastrophizing Scale: User manual. Montreal: McGill University, 2009.

[7] Sullivan, MJL. The communal coping model of pain catastrophzing: Clinical and research implications. Can Psychol 2012;53(1):32.

[8] Wertli MM, Eugster R, Held U, Steurer J, Kofmehl R, Weiser S. Catastrophizing: A prognostic factor for outcome in patients with low back pain: A systematic review. Spine J 2014;14(11):2639-57.

[9] Ayers DC, Franklin PD, Trief PM, Ploutz-Snyder R, Freund D. Psychological attributes of preoperative total joint replacement patients: implications for optimal physical outcome. J Arthroplasty 2004; 19(7):125-30.

[10] Lamé IE, Peters ML, Vlaeyen JW, Kleef MV, Patijn J. Quality of life in chronic pain is more associated with beliefs about pain, than with pain intensity. Eur J Pain 2005;9(1):15-24.

[11] Witvrouw E, Pattyn E, Almqvist KF, Crombez G, Accoe C, Cambier D, et al. Catastrophic thinking about pain as a predictor of length of hospital stay after total knee arthroplasty: A prospective study. Knee Surg Sports Traumatol Arthrosc 2009;17(10):1189-94.

[12] Jacobsen PB and Butler RW. Relation of cognitive coping and catastrophizing to acute pain and analgesic use following breast cancer surgery. J Behav Med 1996;19(1):17-29.

[13] Arnow BA, Blasey CM, Constantino MJ, Robinson R, Hunkeler E, Lee J, et al. Catastrophizing, depression and pain-related disability. Gen Hosp Psychiatry 2011;33(2):150-6.

[14] Severeijns R, Vlaeyen JW, van den Hout MA, Picavet HS. Pain catastrophizing is associated with health indices in musculoskeletal pain: a cross-sectional study in the Dutch community. Health Psychol 2004;23(1):49.

[15] Gibson E, Sabo MT. Can pain catastrophizing be changed in surgical patients? A scoping review. Can J Surgery 2018;61(5):311-8.

[16] Papaioannou M, Skapinakis P, Damigos D, Mavreas V, Broumas G, Palgimesi A. The role of catastrophizing in the prediction of postoperative pain. Pain Med 2009;10(8):1452–9.

[17] Pinto PR, McIntyre T, Almeida A, Araújo-Soares V. The mediating role of pain catastrophizing in the relationship between presurgical anxiety and acute postsurgical pain after hysterectomy. Pain 2012;153(1):218–26.

[18] Granot M and Ferber SG. The roles of pain catastrophizing and anxiety in the prediction of postoperative pain intensity: A prospective study. Clin J Pain 2005;21(5):439–45.

[19] Khan RS, Skapinakis P, Ahmed K, Stefanou DC, Ashrafian H, Darzi A, Athanasiou T. The association between preoperative pain catastrophizing and postoperative pain intensity in cardiac surgery patients. Pain Med 2012;13(6): 820-7.

[20] Helmerhorst GTT, Vranceanu A, Vrahas M, Smith M, Ring D. Risk factors for continued opioid use one to two months after surgery for musculoskeletal trauma. J Bone Joint Surg Am 2014; 96(6):495-9.

[21] Burns LC, Ritvo SE, Ferguson MK, Clarke H, Seltzer ZE, Katz J. Pain catastrophizing as a risk factor for chronic pain after total knee arthroplasty: A systematic review. J Pain Res 2015;8:21.

[22] Vissers MM, Bussmann JB, Verhaar JA, Busschbach JJ, Bierma-Zeinstra SM, Reijman M. Psychological factors affecting the outcome of total hip and knee arthroplasty: A systematic review. Semin Arthritis Rheum 2012;41(4):576-88.

[23] Pavlin DJ, Sullivan MJL, Freund PR, Roesen K. Catastrophizing: A risk factor for postsurgical pain. Clin J Pain 2005;21(1):83–90.

[24] Riddle DL, Wade JB, Jiranek WA, Kong X. Preoperative pain catastrophizing predicts pain outcome after knee arthroplasty. Clin Orthopaedics Relat Res 2010;468(3):798-806.

[25] Wright D, Hoang M, Sofine A, Silva JP, Schwarzkopf R. Pain catastrophizing as a predictor for postoperative pain and opiate consumption in total joint arthroplasty patients. Arch Orthopaedic Trauma Surg 2017;137(12):1623-9.

[26] Darnall BD. Pain psychology and pain catastrophizing in the perioperative setting: A review of impacts, interventions and unmet needs. Hand Clin 2017;32(1):33-9.

[27] den Boer JJ, Oostendorp RA, Beems T, Munneke M, Oerlemans M, Evers AW. A systematic review of bio-psychosocial risk factors for an unfavourable outcome after lumbar disc surgery. Eur Spine J 2006;15(5):527-36.

[28] Cook CE. Clinimetrics corner: the minimal clinically important change score (MCID): A necessary pretense. J Manual Manipul Ther 2008;16(4):82E-3E.

[29] Farrar JT, Young Jr JP, LaMoreaux L, Werth JL, Poole RM. Clinical importance of changes in chronic pain intensity measured on an 11-point numerical pain rating scale. Pain 2001;94(2):149-58.

[30] Kennedy DM, Stratford PW, Robarts S and Gollish JD. Using outcome measure results to facilitate clinical decisions the first year after total hip arthroplasty. J Orthopaedic Sports Phys Ther 2011;41(4):232-40.

[31] Forsythe ME, Dunbar MJ, Hennigar AW, Sullivan MJ, Gross M. Prospective relation between catastrophizing and residual pain following knee arthroplasty: two-year follow-up. Pain Res Manage 2008;13(4):335-41.

[32] Noiseux NO, Callaghan JJ, Clark CR, Zimmerman MB, Sluka KA, Rakel BA. Preoperative predictors of pain following total knee arthroplasty. J Arthroplasty 2014;29(7):1383-7.

[33] Bierke S, Petersen W. Influence of anxiety and pain catastrophizing on the course of pain within the first year after uncomplicated total knee replacement: a prospective study. Arch Orthopaedic Traum Surg 2017; 137(12):1735-42.

[34] Dhurve K, Scholes C, El-Tawil S, Shaikh A, Weng LK, Levin K, et al. Multifactorial analysis of dissatisfaction after primary total knee replacement. Knee 2017;24(4):856-62.

[35] Van Onsem S, Van Der Straeten C, Arnout N, Deprez P, Van Damme G, Victor J. A new prediction model for patient satisfaction after total knee arthroplasty. J Arthroplasty 2016;31(12):2660-7.

[36] Riddle DL, Wade JB, Jiranek WA, Kong X. Preoperative pain catastrophizing predicts pain outcome after knee arthroplasty. Clin Orthopaedics Relat Res 2010;468(3):798-806.

[37] Valdes AM, Doherty SA, Zhang W, Muir KR, Maciewicz RA, Doherty M. Inverse relationship between preoperative radiographic severity and postoperative pain in patients with osteoarthritis who have undergone total joint arthroplasty. Semin Arthritis Rheum 2012;41(4):568-75.

[38] Sabo MT, Roy M. Surgeon identification of pain catastrophizing versus the Pain Catastrophizing Scale in orthopaedic patients after routine surgical consultation. Can J Surg 2019;62(4):265-9.

[39] Fisher DA, Dierckman B, Watts MR, Davis K. Looks good but feels bad: factors that contribute to poor results after total knee arthroplasty. J Arthroplasty 2007;6(Suppl 2):39-42.

In: Pain Management
Editors: J Merrick and M Morad ISBN: 978-1-68507-493-7

Chapter 3

EXERCISE THERAPY FOR MUSCULOSKELETAL PAIN AMONG OFFICE WORKERS

Mothna Mohammed Abdulameer**, MSc,
Ali Kareem Finteel, PhD
and Sajjad Kareem Flayyih, MSc
Department of Physical Education and Sport Sciences,
AlSafwa University College, Karbala, Iraq

ABSTRACT

Sitting for a long time and absence of physical activity, could be considered as the main reasons for musculoskeletal pain. This pain could affect daily life of office workers and for sure it would have a negative impact on their working efficacy. This pain could be followed by secondary problems such as obesity, knee pain and maybe psychological issues. In this regards, there are different types of therapy suggested for

* ***Correspondence:*** Mothna Mohammed Abdulameer, MSc, Department of Physical Education and Sport Sciences, AlSafwa University College, Karbala, Iraq.
Email: muthanamuh8@gmail.com.

this purpose. Exercise therapy is one of the most common therapy suggested for prevention and therapy of musculoskeletal pain. This review paper has tried to make a collection from novel and new methods of exercise therapy presented for office workers, who sit for long time. Among those papers, English publications released from 2012 to 2020 are included. The main key words were including "office workers," "musculoskeletal pain," "exercise," "therapy." The results showed that, home based/office based exercise are the most feasible kinds of exercise therapy, as those are cost effective and easy to do.

INTRODUCTION

Active life style is slowly being replaced with sedentary life style and the main reason could be related to the developing of countries and demands of societies (1). Office workers are a group of individuals who are forced to work in sitting position for long time and they do not have enough time to perform a regular pattern of physical activity (2,3).

The main effect of this sedentary life style is directly on physical and physiological aspects of office workers (4). Musculoskeletal pain (MP) is the most common symptom of this unhealthy lifestyle and usually defined as a set of physical or chemical disorders in one or more group of muscles, tendons, joint, nerves or any part of the body that supports the spine and limbs which influenced by anthropometric properties like age, gender or body mass index (5). It could be including a wide range of pain such as low back pain, neck pain, shoulder pain and wrist pain. For sure, those pains can affect the performance of office workers (6). Pain and swelling in the affected areas of the body are the main consequences of musculoskeletal disorders, which in turn can reduce people's daily quality of life (7, 8).

There are different packages of therapy suggested for office workers to prevent or treatment of musculoskeletal pain/discomfort. Some of those therapies such as using medicine has some side effects and some of those such as physiotherapy or occupational therapy is not cost effective, unless the person is in a risky level of pain.

The novelty of this paper is related to the selected papers, as they have suggested feasible exercises, easy to do in office/home. The main purpose of this paper is to introduce an easy and cost effective guideline for the office workers to prevention and treatment of musculoskeletal pain, if it was related to sedentary life style and longtime sitting.

OUR REVIEW

In this narrative review, published papers in English language from 2012-2020 are presented. Keywords including "office workers," "musculoskeletal pain," "exercise," "therapy" and Scopus, PubMed, Google Scholar, Cochrane, and Web of Science were selected as databases. We just focused on papers with home/office based exercise training for musculoskeletal disorder/discomfort/pain among office workers who sit and work at least for eight hours. Among 114 selected papers, finally seven papers were selected based on our defined criteria.

FINDINGS

The main causes of MP in the workplace among office workers are pain due to musculoskeletal disorders in the neck, back, and shoulders (9). Advances in technology have affected the way the office worker accomplish their job and approximately, 50 percent are working with activities that required significant time using the mouse and keyboard. It has been reported that increasing the low back, shoulders, and neck pain is associated with changes in work postures and job duties that can lead to large economic burdens by harming the gross domestic product. Musculoskeletal pain following excessive computer work and incorrect posture can cause symptoms such as pain or tingling/numbness, and often progress to chronic nature.

Table 1. Selected works done related to office/home based exercises for office workers

	Authors/year	Title	Method	Conclusion
1	Shariat A, Tamrin SBM, Arumugam M, Danaee M, Ramasamy R. (2016). (15)	Office exercise training to reduce and prevent the occurrence of musculoskeletal disorders among office workers: a hypothesis.	Introduce an office based package of exercise training based on the American College of Sports Medicine, Williams and Mackenzie suggestions.	This package is able to increase the flexibility and strength of trunk muscles
2	Justesen JB, Søgaard K, Dalager T, Christensen JR, Sjøgaard G. (2017). (16)	The effect of intelligent physical exercise training on sickness presenteeism and absenteeism among office workers	Determine the effect of a one -year exercise training among office workers	Exercise training can improve presenteeism and decrease absenteeism of office workers
3	Shariat A, Lam ET, Kargarfard M, Tamrin S, Danaee M. (2017). (17)	The application of a feasible exercise training program in the office setting	Forty healthy office workers apart from suffering from any sub-clinical symptoms of muscle and joint	The exercise training program can MP and improve the ROM or flexibility of the office workers.
4	Metcalfe RS, Atef H, Mackintosh K, McNarry M, Ryde G, Hill DM, Vollaard NB. (2020). (18)	Time-efficient and computer-guided sprint interval exercise training for improving health in the workplace: a randomized mixed-methods feasibility study in office-based employees	Twenty-five office-workers completed a 6-week REHIT intervention unsupervised in their workplace, or acted as a nonintervention control	REHIT could be implemented as a feasible, effective and acceptable exercise intervention in a workplace setting

	Authors/year	Title	Method	Conclusion
5	Arslan SS, Alemdaroğlu İ, Karaduman AA, Yilmaz ÖT. (2019). (19)	The effects of physical activity on sleep quality, job satisfaction, and quality of life in office workers.	One group performed regular physical activity for at least eight weeks, and another group did not do any regular physical activity.	Regular physical activity could is useful to improve the quality of life.
6	Pereira M, Comans T, Sjøgaard G, Straker L, Melloh M, O'leary S, Johnston V. (2019). (20)	The impact of workplace ergonomics and neck-specific exercise versus ergonomics and health promotion interventions on office worker productivity: A cluster-randomized trial	Tailored workstation ergonomics intervention, followed by workplace neck-specific exercises	This tailored package was effective on health-related productivity loss among office workers
7	Johnston V, Gane EM, Brown W, Vicenzino B, Healy GN, Gilson N, Smith MD. (2019). (21)	Feasibility and impact of sit-stand workstations with and without exercise in office workers at risk of low back pain: A pilot comparative effectiveness trial.	Sit-stand workstation and advice with progressive resistance exercise training for 4-weeks.	Sit-stand workstation was an effective way on reducing LBP.

Physical activity in office workers

Physical activity is an essential part of a healthy lifestyle (10) and is an integral part of the proper functioning of the musculoskeletal system (11). Stiffness and weakness in the joints and muscles are affected by the absence of exercise. People with sedentary lifestyles lose both muscle strength and flexibility, both of which are vital for physical fitness as well as maintaining normal posture (12). Regular exercise nourishes the spinal discs, soft tissues and ligaments. In addition, sitting in an office chair for a long time can cause or worsen existing pain problems. Regular exercise improves nutrition of the spinal discs, soft tissues and ligaments.

Exercise therapy for office workers

However, there is conflicting scientific evidence for exercise therapy related to MP. In a recent systematic study, the effectiveness and safety of exercise therapy have been shown to improve flexibility, strength, and performance, as well as reduce the level of pain (13). From mild physical activity to strenuous exercise or multimodal exercises, the type and intensity of exercise diverse. The type and intensity of exercise varies from mild general physical activity to strenuous exercise and multimodal exercises. Aerobic exercise is as one of the best type of exercise therapy for MP, but it is not easy to do in office/home (14). So, a series of exercise training including flexibility and strength training could be useful.

CONCLUSION

A summary of findings is shown in table 1, which shows that, office/based exercise therapy could be considered as a tailored therapy with office workers with MSP and efficiency of this way is highlighted in previous works clearly. There is still a lack about different pattern of office/home based exercise therapy for MSP and it would be the role of future researches. Those exercises could be divided in aerobic and anaerobic or aerobic and resistance, etc.

REFERENCES

[1] Shariat A, Tamrin SBM, Arumugam M, Danaee M, Ramasamy R. Musculoskeletal disorders and their relationship with physical activities among office workers: A review. Malay J Public Health Med 2016;16(1):62-74.

[2] Mörl F, Bradl I. Lumbar posture and muscular activity while sitting during office work. J Electromyogr Kinesiol 2013;23(2):362–8.

[3] Shariat A, Mohd Tamrin SB, Arumugam M, Danaee M, Ramasamy R. Office exercise training to reduce and prevent the occurrence of musculoskeletal disorders among office workers: A hypothesis. Malays J Med Sci 2016;23(4):54-8.

[4] Coggon D, Ntani G, Palmer KT, Felli VE, Harari R, Barrero LH, et al. Disabling musculoskeletal pain in working populations: Is it the job, the person, or the culture? Pain 2013;154(6):856–63.

[5] Madeleine P. On functional motor adaptations: from the quantification of motor strategies to the prevention of musculoskeletal disorders in the neck–shoulder region. Acta Physiol (Oxf) 2010;199:1–46.

[6] Chung YC, Hung CT, Li SF, Lee HM, Wang SG, Chang SC, et al. Risk of musculoskeletal disorder among Taiwanese nurses cohort: a nationwide population-based study. BMC Musculoskelet Disord 2013;14(1):144.

[7] Nag PK. Musculoskeletal disorders: Office menace. In: Nag PK. Office buildings. New York: Springer, 2019:105–26.

[8] Calik BB, Yagci N, Oztop M, Caglar D. Effects of risk factors related to computer use on musculoskeletal pain in office workers. Int J Occup Saf Ergon 2020 May 06:1–18.

[9] Charles LE, Ma CC, Burchfiel CM, Dong RG. Vibration and ergonomic exposures associated with musculoskeletal disorders of the shoulder and neck. Saf Health Work 2018;9(2):125–32.

[10] Ghannadi S, Amouzegar A, Amiri P, Karbalaeifar R, Tahmasebinejad Z, Kazempour-Ardebili S. Evaluating the effect of knowledge, attitude, and practice on self-management in type 2 diabetic patients on dialysis. J Diabetes Res 2016;2016:3730875.

[11] Nawrocka A, Niestrój-Jaworska M, Mynarski A, Polechonski J. Association between objectively measured physical activity and musculoskeletal disorders, and perceived work ability among adult, middle-aged and older women. Clin Interv Aging 2019;14:1975.

[12] Alsufiany MB, Lohman EB, Daher NS, Gang GR, Shallan AI, Jaber HM. Non-specific chronic low back pain and physical activity: A comparison of postural control and hip muscle isometric strength: A cross-sectional study. Medicine (Baltimore) 2020;99(5):e18544.

[13] Lim K-T, Shin B-C, Park IH, Park SY, Hwang M-S. Daoyin exercise therapy for low back pain: A systematic review. J Korea Manual Med Spin Nerv 2018;13(1):23–33.

[14] Booth J, Moseley GL, Schiltenwolf M, Cashin A, Davies M, Hübscher M. Exercise for chronic musculoskeletal pain: a biopsychosocial approach. Musculoskeletal Care 2017;15(4):413–21.

[15] Shariat A, Tamrin SBM, Arumugam M, Danaee M, Ramasamy R. Office exercise training to reduce and prevent the occurrence of musculoskeletal disorders among office workers: a hypothesis. Malays J Med Sci 2016;23(4):54-8.

[16] Justesen JB, Søgaard K, Dalager T, Christensen JR, Sjøgaard G. The effect of intelligent physical exercise training on sickness presenteeism and absenteeism among office workers. J Occup Environ Med 2017;59(10):942–8.

[17] Shariat A, Lam ETC, Kargarfard M, Tamrin SBM, Danaee M. The application of a feasible exercise training program in the office setting. Work 2017;56(3):421-8

[18] Metcalfe RS, Atef H, Mackintosh K, McNarry M, Ryde G, Hill DM, et al. Time-efficient and computer-guided sprint interval exercise training for improving health in the workplace: a randomised mixed-methods feasibility study in office-based employees. BMC Public Health 2020;20(1):1–13.

[19] Arslan SS, Alemdaroglu I, Karaduman AA, Yilmaz ÖT. The effects of physical activity on sleep quality, job satisfaction, and quality of life in office workers. Work 2019;63(1):3–7.

[20] Pereira M, Comans T, Sjøgaard G, Straker L, Melloh M, O'leary S, et al. The impact of workplace ergonomics and neck-specific exercise versus ergonomics and health promotion interventions on office worker productivity: A cluster-randomized trial. Scand J Work Environ Health 2019;45(1):42–52.

[21] Johnston V, Gane EM, Brown W, Vicenzino B, Healy GN, Gilson N, et al. Feasibility and impact of sit-stand workstations with and without exercise in office workers at risk of low back pain: A pilot comparative effectiveness trial. Appl Ergon 2019;76:82–9.

In: Pain Management
Editors: J Merrick and M Morad
ISBN: 978-1-68507-493-7

Chapter 4

POST STROKE: NEUROREHABILITATION FOR REDUCTION OF PAIN

Mothna Mohammed Abdulameer**, MSc,
Mohammed Hassan Abbas, PhD
and Ebtihal Hasan Abdulameer, MSc
Department of Physical Education and Sport Sciences,
AlSafwa University College, Karbala, Iraq

ABSTRACT

Pain is considered as a common issue among patients post-stroke. Increasing the spasticity in limbs and absence of enough physical activity boost this issue. Rehabilitation and neurorehabilitation are the most common ways to help patients post stroke. There are different techniques used for neurorehabilitation including functional electrical stimulation and other modalities. This review try to explore recent papers used neurorehabilitataioin techniques to help to the patients post stroke published between 2012 to 2020. Google Scholar, PubMed, Scopus and

* ***Correspondence:*** Mothna Mohammed Abdulameer, MSc, Department of Physical Education and Sport Sciences, AlSafwa University College, Karbala, Iraq. Email: muthanamuh8@gmail.com.

Web of Science were used as source. The keywords were including "stroke," "pain," "spasticity," "rehabilitation," "neurorehabilitation." Functional electrical stimulation (FES) for decreasing the level of pain among patients post stroke was found to have positive effects, if the process of therapy gets started on time. In addition, using FES is a practical way to improve the functional performance of patients post stroke, and the main observed effect was related to their gait performance.

INTRODUCTION

Stroke is a neurological issue that affect limbs and is a reason for spasticity in this group of patients (1, 2). Those patients are not able to do their daily activities and they prefer to stay at home and get far from societies. Long time spasticity and absence of enough physical activity could be a reason for pain in those patients (3, 4). There are different ways to help to the patients post stroke, such as hydrotherapy, physiotherapy, occupational therapy (3, 5, 6). Neurorehabilitation including a series of medical process used to help recovery from a nervous system injury, and improve functional ability of those patients. Using functional electrical stimulation is the most common type of neurorehabilitation for the patients post stroke (7). This study tried to select recent published paper about neurorehabilitation for the patients post stroke with focus on real performance of those patients.

OUR REVIEW

In this review, valuable papers published from 2014-2020 were selected. The main keywords were: stroke, pain, neurorehabilitation and rehabilitation. Duplicates were removed and only papers in English language were considered (see Figure 1).

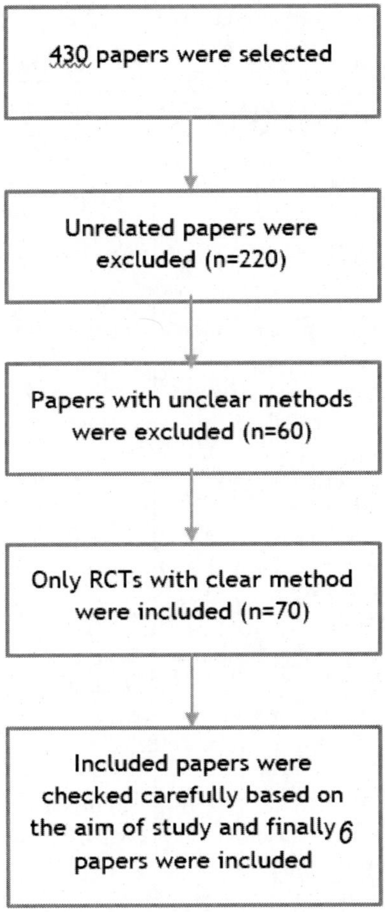

Figure 1. Selection process of articles.

FINDINGS

Findings of this paper are categorized in three main groups and key findings of the previous works are mentioned. A summary of research is shown in Table 1.

Table 1. Selected works related to neurorehabilitation and stroke

	Authors/year	Title	Method	Conclusion
1	Hanger HC, Whitewood, P, Brown G, Ball MC, Harper J, Cox R, Sainsbury R. (2000). (8)	A randomized controlled trial of strapping to prevent post-stroke shoulder pain.	VAS was used to determine the level of pain in shoulder area in patients post stroke.	Late treatment could not be useful to decrease the level of shoulder pain in patients post stroke.
2	Shariat A, Nakhostin Ansari N, Honarpishe R, Moradi V, Hakakzadeh A, Cleland JA, et al. (2019). (9)	Effect of cycling and functional electrical stimulation with linear and interval patterns of timing on gait parameters in patients after stroke: a randomized clinical trial. Disability and rehabilitation	A combination of cycling and FES was used to improve the level of pain and quality of life among patients post stroke.	Neurorehabilitation could be considered as a practical wat to improve the quality of life among patients post stroke.
3	Simons LE, Elman I, Borsook D. (2014). (9)	Psychological processing in chronic pain: a neural systems approach.	Pain neuroscience psychology can enhance our treatment of chronic pain.	Psychological treatments are useful for decreasing the level of pain among patients post stroke.
4	Maier M, Ballester BR, Verschure PF. (2019). (10)	Principles of neurorehabilitation after stroke based on motor learning and brain plasticity mechanisms.	11 principles were compared and analyzed.	Neurorehabilitation combined with motor learning exercise could be effective on spasticity and level of pain.
5	Ciancarelli I, Tonin P, Ciancarelli MGT. (2019). (11)	Effectiveness of intensive neurorehabilitation in obese subacute stroke patients.	Functional recovery and anthropometric characters were determined in patients post stroke.	High BMI could be a reason for decreasing functional recovery.
6	Napoleone D, Silberglied T, L'Abbate G, Fried D. (2019). (11)	The Role of Occupational Therapy in Neurorehabilitation.	Determine the therapeutic use of everyday life activity.	Occupational therapy is useful to improve the function of patients post stroke and decrease the level of pain.

Pain and neurological issues

Nearly 10% of patients have pain after a stroke, which is usually a pain in the form of a hyperaesthesia with burning sensation and aching in affect areas that are numb. Such pain is usually resistant to medical treatment and to the extent that patients do not become without symptoms. Post-stroke shoulder pain is one of the prevalent and disabling post-stroke complications, the prevalence of which can vary from 16 to 80% depending on the type and time of measurement but it is clear that its prevalence increases over time after a stroke.

Reducing the range of motion and decreasing the level of physical activity and quality of life could be considered as the main reasons for this pain. It should be noted that, in some cases, once the stroke occurred among old population, having a chronic pain from past, could be another reason and new condition make it worse.

Stroke

Studies have shown that stroke is one of the leading causes of death and disability. The prevalence of stroke and related disabilities is increasing annually, especially in developing countries (12). Stroke has several negative outcomes including loss of physical performance (walking, daily tasks), social behavior, strength, and postural control that lead to long-term rest and health problems (13). One of the main aims of rehabilitation for this population is to improve their gait and quality of life (14).

Stroke has a plethora of negative effects on patient outcomes such as changes in motor and sensory function resulting in hemiparesis, spasticity, and hemi-neglect. The lifestyle of stroke patients and their families changes, which is associated with decreased performance and activity, substantially activities of daily living (ADLs) (15).

This lifestyle change leads to increment inactivity and complications including falls and subsequent injuries such as imbalance, walking speed, and endurance in patients with stroke (16). In addition, patients after a stroke often depend on other people and assistive devices for ADLs (17, 18). Therefore, improving post-stroke motor outcomes is particularly significant with a focus on neural rehabilitation. Recently, therapeutic interventions concentrate on minimizing complications and coping with limitations, even in simple activities such as walking (10).

Neurorehabilitation

The development of non-invasive brain imaging technologies has increased the perception of neural flexibility, which leads to functional and structural changes in the central nervous system after stroke and rehabilitation (19, 20). Nerve flexibility is the brain's ability to make new neural connections, acquire new functions, and compensate for disorders (21) which are vital for motor recovery after stroke. Different neurorehabilitation schedules are effective for enhancing neural flexibility and improve post-stroke movements, but these interventions show large inter-individual changes in performance due to heterogeneous mechanisms underlying motor recovery among patients (9). Therefore, research is still ongoing to find the combined use of these techniques can improve motor recovery by increasing neural flexibility. It is expected that by the merging of protocols based on various mechanisms, instead of using each treatment method alone, the effects of combined treatment will provide better motor improvement (22).

Conclusion

This review paper tried to determine the available neurorehabilitataion techniques, especially Functional Electrical Stimulation (FES) for decreasing the level of pain among patients post stroke. Based on the previous works, it was shown that, if the process of therapy gets started on time, it could be useful to decrease the severity of pain among this population. In addition, using FES is a practical way to improve the functional performance of patients post stroke, and the main observed effect was related to their gait performance.

REFERENCES

[1] Mochizuki G, Centen A, Resnick M, Lowrey C, Dukelow SP, Scott SH. Movement kinematics and proprioception in post-stroke spasticity: assessment using the Kinarm robotic exoskeleton. J Neuroeng Rehabil 2019;16(1):146.

[2] Scoppettuolo P, Gaspard N, Depondt C, Legros B, Ligot N, Naeije G. Epileptic activity in neurological deterioration after ischemic stroke, a continuous EEG study. Clin Neurophysiol 2019;130(12):2282–6.

[3] Wang M, Zhang Z-L, Wang X, Ji X-Q, Yang Y-Q, Lu X, et al. Clinical trials of acupuncture treatment of post-stroke shoulder pain. Acupunct Res 2019;44(8):605–9.

[4] Duan Y-X, Zhang Z-Q, Luo X-J, Yin J, Xia Y. Randomized controlled trial of internal heat-type acupuncture needle therapy in the treatment of post-stroke shoulder pain. Acupunct Res 2019;44(3):205.

[5] Ghannadi S, Shariat A, Ansari NN, Tavakol Z, Honarpishe R, Dommerholt J, et al. The effect of dry needling on lower limb dysfunction in poststroke survivors. J Stroke Cerebrovasc Dis 2020;29(6):104814.

[6] Tavakol Z, Shariat A, Ghannadi S, Noormohammadpour P, Honarpishe R, Cleland JA, et al. The effect of dry needling on upper and lower limb spasticity in a patient with a brain tumor. Acupunct Med 2019;37(2):133–5.

[7] Shariat A, Ansari NN, Cleland JA, Hakakzadeh A, Kordi R, Kargarfard M. Therapeutic effects of cycling on disability, mobility, and quality of life in patients post stroke. Iran J Public Health 2019;48(2):355.

[8] Hanger HC, Whitewood P, Brown G, Ball MC, Harper J, Cox R, et al. A randomized controlled trial of strapping to prevent post-stroke shoulder pain. Clin Rehabil 2000;14(4):370–80.

[9] Shariat A, Nakhostin Ansari N, Honarpishe R, Moradi V, Hakakzadeh A, Cleland JA, et al. Effect of cycling and functional electrical stimulation with linear and interval patterns of timing on gait parameters in patients after stroke: a randomized clinical trial. Disabil Rehabil 2019 Nov 10;1–7. doi: 10.1080/09638288.2019.1685600.

[10] Maier M, Ballester BR, Verschure PFMJ. Principles of neurorehabilitation after stroke based on motor learning and brain plasticity mechanisms. Front Syst Neurosci 2019;13:74.

[11] Ciancarelli I, Tonin P, Ciancarelli MGT. Effectiveness of intensive neurorehabilitation in obese subacute stroke patients. Funct Neurol 2019;34(1):45–51.

[12] Krishnamurthi R V, Ikeda T, Feigin VL. Global, regional and country-specific burden of ischaemic stroke, intracerebral haemorrhage and subarachnoid haemorrhage: A systematic analysis of the global burden of disease study 2017. Neuroepidemiology 2020;54(2):171–9.

[13] Kwakkel G, Van Wegen EEH, Burridge JH, Winstein CJ, Van Dokkum LEH, Alt Murphy M, et al. Standardized measurement of quality of upper limb movement after stroke: Consensus-based core recommendations from the Second Stroke Recovery and Rehabilitation Roundtable. Neurorehabil Neural Repair 2019;33(11):951–8.

[14] Shariat A, Najafabadi MG, Ansari NN, Cleland JA, Singh MAF, Memari A-H, et al. The effects of cycling with and without functional electrical stimulation on lower limb dysfunction in patients post-stroke: A systematic review with meta-analysis. NeuroRehabilitation 2019;44(3):389–412.

[15] Shilpy PS. Functional outcome of stroke patients after two weeks physiotherapy management at a selected hospital. Dissertation. Dhaka: Bangladesh Health Professions Institute, Faculty of Medicine, 2018.

[16] Simpson LA, Miller WC, Eng JJ. Effect of stroke on fall rate, location and predictors: A prospective comparison of older adults with and without stroke. PLoS One 2011;6(4):e19431.

[17] Hori H, Sonoda S, Watanabe M, Okuyama Y, Okamoto S, Okazaki H. Relationship between change in ADL during two weeks from admission and ADL at discharge in post-stroke patients admitted to Kaifukuki rehabilitation wards. Japan Compr Rehab Sci 2019;10:82–7.

[18] Ranner M, Guidetti S, von Koch L, Tham K. Experiences of participating in a client-centred ADL intervention after stroke. Disabil Rehabil 2019;41(25):3025–33.

[19] Dimyan MA, Cohen LG. Neuroplasticity in the context of motor rehabilitation after stroke. Nat Rev Neurol 2011;7(2):76–85.

[20] Kleim JA, Jones TA. Principles of experience-dependent neural plasticity: implications for rehabilitation after brain damage. J Speech Lang Hear Res 2008, 51(1):S225-39.

[21] Pekna M, Pekny M, Nilsson M. Modulation of neural plasticity as a basis for stroke rehabilitation. Stroke 2012;43(10):2819–28.

[22] Raffin E, Hummel FC. Restoring motor functions after stroke: multiple approaches and opportunities. Neuroscientist 2018;24(4):400–16.

In: Pain Management
Editors: J Merrick and M Morad ISBN: 978-1-68507-493-7

Chapter 5

ATHLETES: THE EFFECT OF PHYSICAL PAIN ON LEVEL OF DEPRESSION AND STATIC BALANCE

Hossein Mafi, MSc and Abdollah Fallahi*, MSc
[1]Department of Motor Behavior, Faculty of Physical Education and Sport Science, University of Tehran, Tehran, Iran

ABSTRACT

To determine the effects of physical pain, on level of depression and static balance of athletes, who has injured during their exercise trainings, is a vital point. For sure, any type of pain, can affect mood and performance. In this review paper, the authors try to collect recent research in this area. There are not many publications with this topic, but the authors of this paper, tried to highlight the importance of research in this field. The published papers in English from 2014 to 2020 were selected and reviewed. The keyword were pain, depression, balance, athletes and injuries. Google Scholar, Web of Science, PubMed and Scopus were the sources for data collection. We found that there is a direct connection among pain, static balance and depression in athletes.

* Corresponding Author's Email: abdollah.fallahii@yahoo.com.

INTRODUCTION

Any injury in the lower back could affect the balance of athletes, but it is not clear if the mechanism of that injury is the reason for the physical pain. In addition, it is not clear if the painful injuries in the upper body can affect the balance of athletes. In 2018, Farahbakhsh et al. (1) showed that neck pain and low back pain among athletes could affect their function. Absence of neuromuscular coordination following the injury and the physical pain could be the reason for this disability. It is shown that, there is a relationship between depression and negative behaviors among athletes, especially related to pain (2). Long-term exercise trainings, chronic and acute pains and the stress and pressures related to the competitions, could be the main reasons for depression and it can have a negative effect on physical performance, especially neuromuscular coordination of athletes. As it was suggested by Shariat et al. (3), attention to the physical and emotional fitness of individuals in any position and any occupations with different tasks is essential. Athletes are a group of individuals where their job is doing exercise (3). We are aware about the lack of research done with focus on all those parameters, but we tried to collect the related papers to attract researchers to work in this field of research.

OUR STUDY

In this paper, previous publications in this field from 2014-2020, were selected. The selection criteria was based on the key words pain, depression, balance, athletes and injuries in the English language. In the start we had the plan to select only randomized linical trials (RCTs), but due to the lack of accurate research within this topic, we included any published paper in Google Scholar, Web of Science, PubMed and Scopus that followed academic patterns of research methods (see Figure 1). One of the researchers tried to search in different databases and the other researcher selected the most related among them. The method of selection is shown in PRISMA flow diagram (see Figure 1).

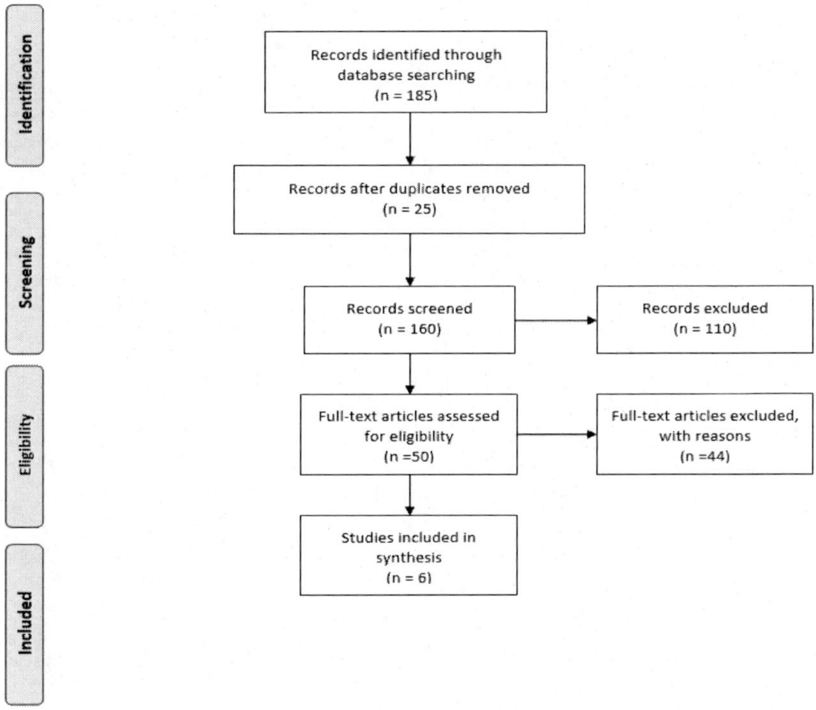

Figure 1. PRISMA flow diagram.

FINDINGS

After 185 papers were selected, we found that 25 papers were duplicated, so we removed those from our collection. Afterwards, again 110 papers were excluded, because they were not focused on our main aim and finally 44 paper were excluded as those papers did not have a very clear method or had lack of justification. A summary of selected papers is shown in Table 1.

Table 1. Selected papers focused on physical pain, depression and static balance in athletes (N = 6)

	Authors	Year of publication	Title	Method	Summary
1	Konietzny K, Chehadi O, Levenig C, Kellmann M, Kleinert J, Mierswa T, Hasenbring MI. (2)	2019	Depression and suicidal ideation in high-performance athletes suffering from low back pain: The role of stress and pain-related thought suppression	159 athletes with low back pain were assessed for depression.	Athletes with higher level of pain, experienced more depression.
2	Belz J, Heidari J, Levenig C, Hasenbring M, Kellmann M, Kleinert J. (4)	2018	Stress and risk for depression in competitive athletes suffering from back pain–Do age and gender matter?.	Among 154 athletes, stress risk and disability was determined.	There was a relationship among depression, pain and disability.
3	Gajsar H, Titze C, Levenig C, Kellmann M, Heidari J, Kleinert J, Hasenbring MI. (5)	2019	Psychological pain responses in athletes and non-athletes with low back pain: Avoidance and endurance matter.	In 173 athletes, the responses of physiological pain to low back pain was determined.	It was shown that, athlete with low back pain, experienced different level of physiological pain
4	Schmidt H, Pedersen TL, Junge T, Engelbert R, Juul-Kristensen B. (6)	2017	Hypermobility in adolescent athletes: pain, functional ability, quality of life, and musculoskeletal injuries	Level of mobility, function and pain was determined among participants.	Hypermobility could be a reason for pain and it is in relation with function.
5	Appiah-Dwomoh E K, Müller S, Mayer F. (7)	2019	Is there an association between variables of static and dynamic postural control in adolescent athletes with back pain?	In 128 athletes, the association between back pain and static balance was determined.	In spite of previous works, this study did not show any relationship between back pain and static balance.
6	San-Antolín M, Rodríguez-Sanz D, López-López D, Romero-Morales, C, Carbajales-Lopez J, Becerro-de-Bengoa-Vallejo, R, Calvo-Lobo C. (8)	2020	Depression levels and symptoms in athletes with chronic gastrocnemius myofascial pain: A case-control study	50 athletes were tested for depression and gastrocnemius myofascial pain.	Higher level of depression was seen in athletes with gastrocnemius myofascial pain.

Physical pain in athletes

There is a wide range of pain among athletes. That pain could be related to the injuries that happened during competition or exercise or it could be related to the chronic injuries that happened related to the repeated movements and nature of their sport (9, 10). The type of pain could also be related to the kinanthropometric attributes of them, that it is different in various sports and genders as well (11). In selected papers, it was showed that, once the athletes are in the competition season, the prevalence of acute injuries occured more than other seasons. Ankle injury was one of the most common injuries in different sports, where the athletes used their lower limbs more than upper limbs, such as football (12). Following that pain, their balance could be affected and it would also affect their performance. There are different ways suggested to use for recovery purposes, such as massage or using NSAIDs (13, 14).

Depression in athletes

Maybe at the first look, there is not any relationship between pain and depression in athletes. But once we look more deeply, we can find it is related. Once an acute or chronic injury happens in athletes, following that injury, pain will appear. That pain would be the reason for their disability or dysfunction. In selected papers, it was shown that the physical pain and being far from exercise training, had a negative effect on their mood and they could feel depressed. This depression could be increased by the level of hormones in response to pain (15, 16). Different types of exercise training and various sports have different effects on depression of athletes. For example, it is shown that aerobic exercise trainings could be more effective on depression in comparison with an aerobic exercise training (17).

Static balance in athletes

There are many parameters that can affect the static balance of athletes and the most important is neuromuscular coordination (18). There is a relation between pain and static balance. Moreno et al. (19) showed that spine stability and strength of muscle in the spine area are related with static balance of athletes. It was mentioned that, once the athletes have any pain in this area, it can directly affect their neuromuscular coordination and it has a negative effect on their balance (19).

Review of selected papers in our study confirmed this theory and hypermobility was considered as another reason for physical pain in the athlete. For sure that pain can affect their static balance as well.

CONCLUSION

As it is summarized in this study, there is a direct connection between pain, static balance and depression in athletes. For sure we cannot stop their exercise training or decrease the intensity of their exercises, but we can follow the related periodization in their trainings and also use the correct recovery techniques in different seasons of training. Athletes can suffer from physical pain and decreased level of health, but if coaches become aware of symptoms of pain and depression, they could be able to determine it in early stages. Having regular neuromuscular coordination trainings, is another way to keep their balance at an acceptable level.

REFERENCES

[1] Farahbakhsh F, Akbari-Fakhrabadi M, Shariat A, Cleland JA, Farahbakhsh F, Seif-Barghi T, et al. Neck pain and low back pain in relation to functional disability in different sport activities. J Exerc Rehabil 2018;14(3):509.

[2] Konietzny K, Chehadi O, Levenig C, Kellmann M, Kleinert J, Mierswa T, et al. Depression and suicidal ideation in high-performance athletes suffering from low

back pain: The role of stress and pain-related thought suppression. Eur J Pain 2019;23(6):1196–208.

[3] Shariat A. Occupational physical and emotional fitness. Work 2018;59(3):463-7.

[4] Belz J, Heidari J, Levenig C, Hasenbring M, Kellmann M, Kleinert J. Stress and risk for depression in competitive athletes suffering from back pain–Do age and gender matter? Eur J Sport Sci 2018;18(7):1029–37.

[5] Gajsar H, Titze C, Levenig C, Kellmann M, Heidari J, Kleinert J, et al. Psychological pain responses in athletes and non-athletes with low back pain: Avoidance and endurance matter. Eur J Pain 2019;23(9):1649–62.

[6] Schmidt H, Pedersen TL, Junge T, Engelbert R, Juul-Kristensen B. Hypermobility in adolescent athletes: pain, functional ability, quality of life, and musculoskeletal injuries. J Orthop Sports Phys Ther 2017;47(10):792–800.

[7] Appiah-Dwomoh EK, Müller S, Mayer F. Is there an association between variables of static and dynamic postural control in adolescent athletes with back pain? German J Exec Sport Res 2019;49(2):150–5.

[8] San-Antolín M, Rodríguez-Sanz D, López-López D, Romero-Morales C, Carbajales-Lopez J, Becerro-de-Bengoa-Vallejo R, et al. Depression levels and symptoms in athletes with chronic gastrocnemius myofascial pain: A case-control study. Phys Ther Sport 2020;43:166-72.

[9] McCarty LP. Approach to medial elbow pain in the throwing athlete. Curr Rev Musculoskelet Med 2019;12(1):30–40.

[10] Villavicencio AT, Hernández TD, Burneikiene S, Thramann J. Neck pain in multisport athletes. J Neurosurg Spine 2007;7(4):408–13.

[11] Shariat A, Shaw BS, Kargarfard M, Shaw I, Lam ETC. Kinanthropometric attributes of elite male Judo, Karate and Taekwondo athletes. Rev Brasi Med Esport 2017;23(4).

[12] Hunt KJ, Hurwit D, Robell K, Gatewood C, Botser IB, Matheson G. Incidence and epidemiology of foot and ankle injuries in elite collegiate athletes. Am J Sports Med 2017;45(2):426–33.

[13] Kargarfard M, Lam ETC, Shariat A, Shaw I, Shaw BS, Tamrin SBM. Efficacy of massage on muscle soreness, perceived recovery, physiological restoration and physical performance in male bodybuilders. J Sports Sci 2016;34(10):959-65.

[14] O'Connor S, McCaffrey N, Whyte E, Moran K, Lacey P. Nonsteroidal anti-inflammatory drug use, knowledge, and behaviors around their use and misuse in Irish collegiate student-athletes. Phys Sportsmed 2019;47(3):318–22.

[15] Case JC. Psychometric properties of the college athlete psychological screening tool: validation of the depression and anxiety subscales. Dissertation. Bowling Green, KY: Western Kentucky University, 2020.

[16] Tahtinen RE, Kristjansdottir H. The influence of anxiety and depression symptoms on help-seeking intentions in individual sport athletes and non-athletes: the role of gender and athlete status. J Clin Sport Psychol 2018;13(1):134–51.

[17] Kianian T, Kermansaravi F, Saber S, Aghamohamadi F. The impact of aerobic and anaerobic exercises on the level of depression, anxiety, stress and happiness of non-athlete male. Zahed J Res Med Sci 2018;20(1):1–6.

[18] DiCesare CA, Montalvo A, Foss KDB, Thomas SM, Hewett TE, Jayanthi NA, et al. Sport specialization and coordination differences in multisport adolescent female basketball, soccer, and volleyball athletes. J Athl Train 2019;54(10):1105–14.

[19] Moreno Catalá M, Schroll A, Laube G, Arampatzis A. Muscle strength and neuromuscular control in low-back pain: elite athletes versus general population. Front Neurosci 2018;12:436.

In: Pain Management
Editors: J Merrick and M Morad
ISBN: 978-1-68507-493-7

Chapter 6

OFFICE WORKERS: PHYSICAL AND SOCIAL PAIN AND ITS RELATION WITH MOTOR DYSFUNCTION

Sanaz Faraji*[*], *PhD and Zahra Nasiri, MSc
Department of Motor Behavior, Faculty of Physical Education and Sport Science, University of Tehran, Tehran, Iran

ABSTRACT

Office workers are a group of individuals, who sit for a long time and also lack of physical activity. Low back pain, neck pain and shoulder pain are the most common types of pain among this group. Working stress, absence of enough care about employers, and anxiety related to their position are the reason for their social pain. A combination of social and physical pain could be the main reason for motor dysfunction among them. Here we have tried to collect the recent papers focused on this topic published from 2016 to 2020. The main aim of this review was to determine the reasons and level of pain among office workers to attract future researchers to find a solution for prevention or treatment. However, currently there are some solutions that we will mention in this paper.

[*] Corresponding Author's Email: faraji.snz79@yahoo.com.

INTRODUCTION

In the current situation of the world with Covid-19, most of the occupations and tasks are converted to home based or office based works (1). Individuals will sit at home or in their office and do their tasks with personal computer/lap top (2). This long time sitting and working with their computer, makes them prone for musculoskeletal disorders such as neck, shoulder and lower back pain (3, 4). People are worried about their salary and future of their job and cannot predict the future of their work and this stress and anxiety, makes for a social pain (5, 6). For sure, this physical and social pain, can affect their performance and efficiency of the company. Once they experience pain for a long period of time, it can affect their daily mood as well. A mixture of those issues, can lead to physical and psychological problems. Depression could be considered as one of the most common issues among individuals, who suffer from social pain (7). Motor dysfunction and lack of concentration in their tasks, is another negative outcome related to physical pain (8, 9). Motor dysfunction is not only related to the learning process, but also refers to balance and coordination. Because of the pain in their body, especially in their lower back area, they cannot sit properly and they will lose their motivation for improving the company or employer. In this review, we tried to summarize papers related to physical and social pain, which can that lead to motor dysfunction among office workers.

OUR STUDY

English papers focused on social and physical pain were selected from PubMed, Scopus, Google Scholar and Web of Science and checked if it was related to office workers or computer based workers. The year of publication was between 2016-2020, as we wanted to summarize the recent papers published in this area of knowledge. The selection is shown in Figure 1.

Table 1. Selected works related to social pain and physical on motor function in office workers

	Authors/year	Title	Method	Conclusion
1	Andersen LL et al. 2010 (10)	Effect of physical exercise interventions on musculoskeletal pain in all body regions among office workers: A one-year randomized controlled trial	A single blind RCT among 549 office Workers, focused on neck and shoulder.	Resistance exercise had a positive effect on neck and shoulder
2	Lidegaard M et al. 2013 (11)	Effect of Brief Daily Resistance Training on Occupational Neck/Shoulder Muscle Activity in Office Workers with Chronic Pain: Randomized Controlled Trial	30 female office workers with chronic neck and shoulder pain	Level of pain in neck and shoulder was affected by resistance training.
3	Kawaharada M et al. 2013 (12)	Depression prevention program for workers of private companies: A randomized controlled trial	93 workers of two private companies participated in educational program related to stress.	The educational program was useful for coping and managing stress.
4	Kim TH et al. 2015 (13)	The effects of the Core programme on pain at rest, movement-induced and secondary pain, active range of motion, and proprioception in female office workers with chronic low back pain: a randomized controlled trial	53 participants with chronic low back pain	Core training is effective on chronic low back pain.
5	Clevers E et al. 2020 (14)	Gastrointestinal symptoms in office workers are predicted by psychological distress and short sleep duration.	1002 office employees who had gastrointestinal symptoms	Short sleep and long time working could be the reason for gastrointestinal symptoms

Table 1. (Continued)

	Authors/year	Title	Method	Conclusion
6	Aryaie M et al. 2017 (15)	Psychosocial and work-related factors associated with musculoskeletal pain among office workers in Gorgan, North of Iran	675 office staff was included to be interviewed from the 18 occupational sectors focused on psychosocial and work-related factors.	Long time sitting and absence of physical activity were considered as the main reasons for Psychosocial and work-related issues.
7	Shariat A et al. 2018 (16)	Effects of stretching exercise training and ergonomic modifications on musculoskeletal discomforts of office workers: a randomized controlled trial	142 office workers with neck, shoulders, and lower back pain.	Exercise and ergonomic modification were effective to decrease the level of pain in neck, shoulder and lower back.

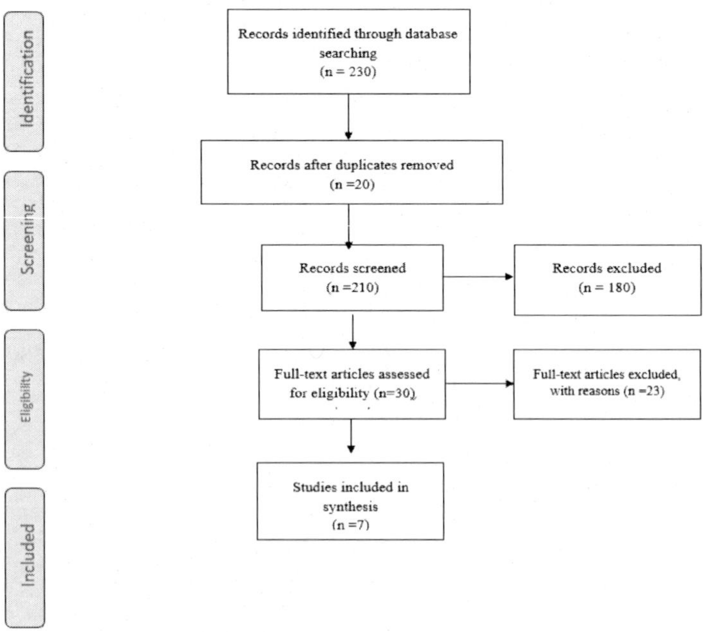

Figure 1. PRISMA 2009 flow diagram.

FINDINGS

After analyzing the selected papers (n = 7), among 230 papers, it was found that, there was a direct relationship between physical and social pain and motor dysfunction in office workers. Long time sitting and lack of physical activity were the main reasons for those pain and motor dysfunction. There were some suggested solutions, about office-based exercises and some techniques for psychological purposes, but there is a need for a package program of treatment and prevention related to physical and social pain, specified for office workers. Findings showed that, the most common type of physical pain was seen in wrist, lower back, neck and shoulder, especially among office workers who were overweight. The most common types of social pain were the stress of losing job, absence of attention from employers, and absence of a bright working future. All those issues can lead to decrease the level of efficiency among office/computer based workers.

Physical pain in office workers

Prolonged sitting and absence of physical activity can lead to different types of physical pain. Those pains have a wide variety and can include wrist, neck, shoulder and lower back. Severity of that pain is also related to the age and body mass index of individuals (2). Different studies have demonstrated the effect of ergonomic modification to prevent from physical pain. As it was mentioned by Shariat et al. (17) there are different ways to determine the physical pain among office workers with the Cornell questionnaire introduced as one of the easiest ways (17). One of the problems related to physical pain is related to the efficiency of office workers. Once they feel the pain, they need to go for rest and it has a huge cost not only for the company, but also for the government. Meanwhile, this pain can lead to motor dysfunction that could be seen in different areas of body. Therefore, it is important to pay attention to the prevention and treatment in early stages.

Social pain in office workers

Today with the Covid-19 situation, we are faced with a new mode of working life. It means all the services and tasks are replaced with digital tasks. This transition has increased stress for any job. Workers and staff are worried about this rapid change and they are not adopted fully. Employers are trying the decrease the number of staff and improve the payments and efficiency. For sure, those changes will make a stress among office workers as well. They cannot predict their future and especially the office workers, who are older, cannot adopt themselves with this new life style (18). In addition, long term working at home, has made them socially isolated. Those changes can make a type of pain, called social pain. Having an emotional fitness is necessary for any occupation and absence of that, can lead to different types of physical and psychological issues (19). That pain not only will affect the emotional performance of office workers, but also their physical performance specially their motor performance.

Motor dysfunction in office workers

Motor function refers to the different types of ability related to learning, maintenance, coordination and posture. Any physical or psychological issue in individuals can lead to motor dysfunction. It means their learning process; neuromuscular coordination and posture will be affected. As it is mentioned above, physical and social pain are the two types of pain seen in office workers that can lead to motor dysfunction (2, 20). Severity of this dysfunction could be related to age of individuals as well. Doing games or activities in groups in the working environment, can prevent motor dysfunction (2). We cannot prevent fully, but with those trainings we can improve the learning and coordination ability in office workers.

Conclusion

As mentioned in the selected papers, occupational and emotional fitness are essential for any job to improve the level of their tasks. Absence of any of those parameters can affect the performance of individual and the company together. Physical and social pains are two types of pain that will occur, once there is lack of emotional and occupational fitness among office workers. Educational programs and having a routine pattern of physical activity could be useful to prevent from it.

References

[1] Shariat A, Hakakzadeh A, Cleland J. Home-based exercise note in Covid-19 quarantine situation for office workers: A commentary. Work 2020;66(2):381-2.

[2] Gardner B, Flint S, Rebar AL, Dewitt S, Quail SK, Whall H, et al. Is sitting invisible? Exploring how people mentally represent sitting. Int J Behav Nutr Phys Act 2019;16(1):85-91.

[3] Shariat A, Cardoso JR, Cleland JA, Danaee M, Ansari NN, Kargarfard M, et al. Prevalence rate of neck, shoulder and lower back pain in association with age, body mass index and gender among Malaysian office workers. Work 2018;60(2):191-9.

[4] Besharati A, Daneshmandi H, Zareh K, Fakherpour A, Zoaktafi M. Work-related musculoskeletal problems and associated factors among office workers. Int J Occup Saf Ergon 2020;26(3):632–8.

[5] Collins JM, Nafziger M. Evaluating financial capability services provided in a workforce development program. J Consum Affair 2019;53(4):1775–96.

[6] Pereira M, Comans T, Sjøgaard G, Straker L, Melloh M, O'leary S, et al. The impact of workplace ergonomics and neck-specific exercise versus ergonomics and health promotion interventions on office worker productivity: A cluster-randomized trial. Scand J Work Environ Health 2019;45(1):42–52.

[7] Majumdar P, Biswas A, Sahu S. COVID-19 pandemic and lockdown: cause of sleep disruption, depression, somatic pain, and increased screen exposure of office workers and students of India. Chronobiol Int 2020; 37(8):1191-200.

[8] Huber J, Lisiński P, Polowczyk A. Reinvestigation of the dysfunction in neck and shoulder girdle muscles as the reason of cervicogenic headache among office workers. Disabil Rehabil 2013;35(10):793–802.

[9] Johnston V, Jull G, Darnell R, Jimmieson NL, Souvlis T. Alterations in cervical muscle activity in functional and stressful tasks in female office workers with neck pain. Eur J Appl Physiol 2008;103(3):253–64.

[10] Andersen LL, Christensen KB, Holtermann A, Poulsen OM, Sjøgaard G, Pedersen MT, et al. Effect of physical exercise interventions on musculoskeletal pain in all body regions among office workers: a one-year randomized controlled trial. Man Ther 2010;15(1):100–4.

[11] Lidegaard M, Jensen RB, Andersen CH, Zebis MK, Colado JC, Wang Y, et al. Effect of brief daily resistance training on occupational neck/shoulder muscle activity in office workers with chronic pain: randomized controlled trial. Biomed Res Int 2013; 26238.

[12] Kawaharada M, Ueda I, Yoshioka E, Hirano M, Ikeno TT, Shindou Y, et al. Depression prevention program for workers of private companies: A randomized controlled trial. Open J Nurs 2013;3(1): 114-21.

[13] Kim TH, Kim E-H, Cho H. The effects of the CORE programme on pain at rest, movement-induced and secondary pain, active range of motion, and proprioception in female office workers with chronic low back pain: a randomized controlled trial. Clin Rehabil 2015;29(7):653–62.

[14] Clevers E, Lutin E, Cornelis J, Van Oudenhove L. Gastrointestinal symptoms in office workers are predicted by psychological distress and short sleep duration. J Psychosom Res 2020;110230.

[15] Aryaie M, Youefi Z, Karimi S, Bagheri D, Bakhsha F, Jafari S Y et al. Psychosocial and work-related factors associated with musculoskeletal pain among office workers in Gorgan, North of Iran. J Clin Bas Res 2017;1(3):8–14.

[16] Shariat A, Cleland JA, Danaee M, Kargarfard M, Sangelaji B, Tamrin SBM. Effects of stretching exercise training and ergonomic modifications on musculoskeletal discomforts of office workers: a randomized controlled trial. Braz J Phys Ther 2018;22(2): 144-153.

[17] Shariat A, Tamrin SBM, Arumugam M, Danaee M, Ramasamy R. Comparative reliability of different instruments used to measure the severity of musculoskeletal disorders in office workers. Work 2016;54(3): 753-8.

[18] Bartik AW, Bertrand M, Cullen ZB, Glaeser EL, Luca M, Stanton CT. How are small businesses adjusting to covid-19? early evidence from a survey. National Bureau of Economic Research 2020.

[19] Shariat A. Occupational physical and emotional fitness. Work 2018;59(3):463-7.

[20] Graven-Nielsen T, Svensson P, Arendt-Nielsen L. Effects of experimental muscle pain on muscle activity and co-ordination during static and dynamic motor function. Electroencephalogr Clin Neurophysiol 1997;105(2):156–64.

In: Pain Management
Editors: J Merrick and M Morad
ISBN: 978-1-68507-493-7

Chapter 7

CORONARY HEART DISEASES: PHYSICAL PAIN AND MOTOR SKILL

Amir Sobh-Rhakhshankhah[1,*], MD and Sanaz Faraji[2], PhD
[1]Sepehr Heart Center, Baharloo Hospital,
Tehran University of Medical Sciences, Tehran, Iran
[2]Department of Motor Behavior, Faculty of Physical Education
and Sport Science, University of Tehran, Tehran, Iran

ABSTRACT

Coronary heart disease (CHD) is considered as one of the most important causes of mortality in the world. Feeling different levels of physical pain and change in motor skill abilities could be happen following CHD. In recent studies, the relationship between physical pain, motor skill abilities and CHD, is not highlighted enough. This paper has tried to focus on this relationship by searching among published papers available in Scopus, PubMed, and Google Scholar from 2010 until 2020. The main reason is to show that, CHD not only affect the physiological parameters

* Corresponding Author's Email: amir.rakhshann@yahoo.com.

of patients, but also is a reason for physical pain and motor skill disability.

INTRODUCTION

The plaques that close the vessels or make it tight cause coronary heart disease (CHD). There are different methods used to diagnose CHD, such as CT scan and MRI. Attention to CHD is important, because it can lead to heart attack (1, 2). There is a need to make some changes in the lifestyle of the patients with CHD, such as stopping smoking and do regular exercise trainings. By being active, having healthy foods and giving up smoking, you can prevent CHD (3).

The person with CHD can feel pain in his/her chest. The patient also will experience weakness in legs or arms, if the vessels are narrowed, and it can affect their motor performance (4, 5). Therefore, attention to the motor skill programs could be important. This chapter has tried to find the recent papers with attention to CHD, physical pain and motor skill disability in patients with CHD.

OUR STUDY

Based on the main aim of this study, we looked at papers published from 2010 until 2020, available in Scopus, PubMed and Google Scholar, with attention to coronary heart disease and its relation with physical pain and motor skills in patients with CHD. Among those papers, seven papers were selected based on the inclusion criteria. It should be noted that, papers that were not in the English language, were not included.

FINDINGS

From the selected papers we observed a direct relationship between lifestyle and CHD. Doing regular physical activity and attention to a healthy diet could prevent CHD. The papers discussed chest pain and weakness in arms and legs affecting motor skills of patients.

Coronary heart disease (CHD)

Coronary heart disease could be considered as a group of disease that includes both heart and vessels. Unfortunately, because of the new and modern lifestyles, especially in developed countries, CHD is an important cause of mortality and disability. High level of elevated low-density lipoprotein cholesterol has a direct relationship with CHD that could be controlled, by changing the lifestyle. It is important to know that, pollution and stress can boost the risk factors of CHD, especially in big cities (6). CHD is preventable, but absence of attention to the diet, physical activity and smoking are the most common habits in developed countries, that are the reasons for CHD. In western countries, the number of mortalities related to CHD has decreased, but the occurrence of CHD is not changed, because of their lifestyle.

Coronary heart disease and physical pain

Chest pain is the most common type of physical pain related to CHD, but it is interesting to know that an association between low back pain and CHD was observed, but it should be noted that there are many studies with opposite opinions in this regard (7). Recently in some studies, it is mentioned that people with spinal pain (low back or neck pain), has a higher prevalence of CHD (8–10). It is mentioned that individuals with musculoskeletal discomforts have higher level of pain spread (11, 12).

Coronary heart disease and motor skills

Motor skill impairment is not reported in direct relationship with CHD, but because of the physical pain created by CHD and especially the weakness of arms and legs, there is a possibility to decrease the ability to do the accurate movements (13, 14). Different types and symptoms of restless leg in relation with CHD are reported. Because of restless leg, most of the individuals reported lack of sleep that could be as a risk factor for CHD. This lack of sleeping and abnormal movements of leg could also be a reason for obesity as another risk factor for CHD (15, 16).

Coronary Heart Disease and Exercise

Different types of exercise trainings could be used to prevent CHD. The patterns of exercise trainings should be done regularly with specific intensities for different age groups (17). Interestingly, there is no data about effectiveness of physical activity on CHD in females who smoke (18). Current suggestions about physical activity are a little different with previous guides, as they suggested that doing physical activity with any intensity is useful for prevention of CHD, but current guides mentioned that the level of intensity should be considered. Regular exercise training, such as hydrotherapy, with lower risk of falling, with focus on neuromuscular coordination and improving the balance in patients is useful (19, 20).

Conclusion

Physical pain, especially in chest area and weakness of limbs are in relation with CHD, that could be prevented or controlled, by cardiac rehabilitation and also following the standard patterns of physical activity. Following a healthy lifestyle, having enough physical activity, and eating healthy foods, are the suggested practical actions to prevent from CHD.

REFERENCES

[1] Williams MC, Moss AJ, Dweck M, Adamson PD, Alam S, Hunter A, et al. Coronary artery plaque characteristics associated with adverse outcomes in the SCOT-HEART study. J Am Coll Cardiol 2019;73(3):291–301.

[2] Plichart M, Celermajer DS, Zureik M, Helmer C, Jouven X, Ritchie K, et al. Carotid intima-media thickness in plaque-free site, carotid plaques and coronary heart disease risk prediction in older adults. The Three-City Study. Atherosclerosis 2011;219(2):917–24.

[3] Stewart RAH, Held C, Krug-Gourley S, Waterworth D, Stebbins A, Chiswell K, et al. Cardiovascular and lifestyle risk factors and cognitive function in patients with stable coronary heart disease. J Am Heart Assoc 2019;8(7):e010641.

[4] de Heer EW, Palacios JE, Adèr HJ, van Marwijk HWJ, Tylee A, van der Feltz-Cornelis CM. Chest pain, depression and anxiety in coronary heart disease: Consequence or cause? A prospective clinical study in primary care. J Psychosom Res 2020;129:109891.

[5] Haasenritter J, Donner-Banzhoff N, Bösner S. Chest pain for coronary heart disease in general practice: Clinical judgement and a clinical decision rule. Br J Gen Pract 2015;65(640):e748–53.

[6] Kargarfard M, Shariat A, Shaw BS, Shaw I, Lam ETC, Kheiri A, et al. Effects of polluted air on cardiovascular and hematological parameters after progressive maximal aerobic exercise. Lung 2015;193(2):275-81.

[7] Vogt MT, Nevitt MC, Cauley JA. Back problems and atherosclerosis: The study of osteoporotic fractures. Spine 1997;22(23):2741–7.

[8] Strine TW, Hootman JM. US national prevalence and correlates of low back and neck pain among adults. Arth Care Res 2007;57(4):656–65.

[9] Fernández-de-las-Peñas C, Alonso-Blanco C, Hernández-Barrera V, Palacios-Ceña D, Jiménez-García R, Carrasco-Garrido P. Has the prevalence of neck pain and low back pain changed over the last 5 years? A population-based national study in Spain. Spine J 2013;13(9):1069–76.

[10] Fernandez M, Ordoñana JR, Hartvigsen J, Ferreira ML, Refshauge KM, Sánchez-Romera JF, et al. Is chronic low back pain associated with the prevalence of coronary heart disease when genetic susceptibility is considered? A co-twin control study of Spanish twins. PLoS One 2016;11(5):e0155194.

[11] Von Korff M, Crane P, Lane M, Miglioretti DL, Simon G, Saunders K, et al. Chronic spinal pain and physical–mental comorbidity in the United States: Results from the national comorbidity survey replication. Pain 2005;113(3):331–9.

[12] Ryan CG, McDonough S, Kirwan JP, Leveille S, Martin DJ. An investigation of association between chronic musculoskeletal pain and cardiovascular disease in the H ealth S urvey for England (2008). Eur J Pain 2014;18(5):740–50.

[13] Miller MS, VanBuren P, LeWinter MM, Lecker SH, Selby DE, Palmer BM, et al. Mechanisms underlying skeletal muscle weakness in human heart failure: alterations in single fiber myosin protein content and function. Circ Heart Fail 2009;2(6):700–6.

[14] Lalani SR, Liu P, Rosenfeld JA, Watkin LB, Chiang T, Leduc MS, et al. Recurrent muscle weakness with rhabdomyolysis, metabolic crises, and cardiac arrhythmia due to bi-allelic TANGO2 mutations. Am J Hum Genet 2016;98(2):347–57.

[15] Walters AS, Rye DB. Review of the relationship of restless legs syndrome and periodic limb movements in sleep to hypertension, heart disease, and stroke. Sleep 2009;32(5):589–97.

[16] Pennestri MH, Montplaisir J, Colombo R, Lavigne G, Lanfranchi PA. Nocturnal blood pressure changes in patients with restless legs syndrome. Neurology 2007;68(15):1213–8.

[17] Kargarfard M, Lam ETC, Shariat A, Asle Mohammadi M, Afrasiabi S, Shaw I, et al. Effects of endurance and high intensity training on ICAM-1 and VCAM-1 levels and arterial pressure in obese and normal weight adolescents. Phys Sportsmed 2016;44(3): 208-16.

[18] Lee I-M, Rexrode KM, Cook NR, Manson JE, Buring JE. Physical activity and coronary heart disease in women: Is no pain, no gain passé? JAMA 2001;285(11):1447–54.

[19] Kargarfard M, Shariat A, Ingle L, Cleland JA, Kargarfard M. Randomized controlled trial to examine the impact of aquatic exercise training on functional capacity, balance, and perceptions of fatigue in female patients with Multiple Sclerosis. Arch Phys Med Rehabil 2018;99(2):234–41.

[20] Michalsen A, Lüdtke R, Bühring M, Spahn G, Langhorst J, Dobos GJ. Thermal hydrotherapy improves quality of life and hemodynamic function in patients with chronic heart failure. Am Heart J 2003;146(4):728–33.

In: Pain Management ISBN: 978-1-68507-493-7
Editors: J Merrick and M Morad

Chapter 8

ATHLETES: SOCIAL PAIN, PHYSICAL PAIN, AND CRIMINAL LAW

Ali Sabzevari, MSc and Sanaz Faraji*, MSc
Department of Criminal Law, Arak Azad University,
Arak and Department of Motor Behavior,
Faculty of Physical Education and Sport Sciences,
University of Tehran, Tehran, Iran

ABSTRACT

Chronic or acute pain is common in athletes, because of the stress of training/injuries. This pain could appear in their physical body or it could experienced in their mind and social life. The outcome of this pain could be shown as their aggressive behaviors during the matches or in their reactions to their family or society. This paper is trying to analyze published papers on this topic. For this aim, we searched papers in Scopus, PubMed and Google Scholar and selected the papers published from 2012 until 2020. We found six papers and showed that, there is not

---

* ***Correspondence:*** Sanaz Faraji, MSc, Department of Motor Behavior, Faculty of Physical Education and Sport Sciences, University of Tehran, Tehran, Iran.
Email: Faraji.snz79@yahoo.com.

a specific guideline or instruction to manage or help the athletes, who suffer from physical and social pain.

INTRODUCTION

Occurrence of pain is a common issue among athletes. Extensive training, stress of competitions and other types of pressure made by their environment are the main reasons for this pain. The physical pain can not only affect their performance, but also create another type of pain called social pain. The athletes with physical pain, cannot sleep well, and cannot participate fully in their training and competition which can make them aggressive and sometimes depressed. Those social pains can affect their relationship with their family and the members of their team. Due to those pains, unexpected behaviors can be observed and managers of team need to be aware about prevention or controlling these behaviors. This review is trying to find available papers published with a focus on this issue and try to find the available solutions for prevention from or solution of this issue.

OUR REVIEW

In this paper we searched Scopus, PubMed, and Google Scholar using selected keywords including pain, physical pain, social pain, law in sport and athletes. We selected English papers published from 2012 to 2020 with a focus on social and physical pain and related laws. Among those papers, six papers were selected and analyzed.

FINDINGS

The six papers claim that athletes are always faced with different types of physical pain and because of that physical pain, their mind can also be affected. Sometimes they will get so aggressive or sometimes they display depression. As they are worried about their competitions and coaches, they will not refer to the physician legally and they try to relieve their pain using steroids. Here we have summarized the findings from the six papers in three different sections including: physical pain, social pain and pain and law.

Physical pain

Athletes normally face with physical challenges during their exercise training or competitions. They have to try to control their physical movements and tasks, in contact or noncontact sports. So, they are prone to injuries and pressure in different parts of their body, such as the lower back (1, 2). It should be noted that it seems that the feeling the pain in athletes is different from normal people, as they face pain but continue their training or competition and it seems that the threshold of pain is changed among athletes. Some of the papers claim that after an intense bouts of exercise training the perception of pain will decrease. Endurance exercise is known to promote sustained anti-nociceptive effects, potentially mediated through central opioidergic neurotransmission. Pain is a natural protective mechanism to help individuals to prevent injuries and in general, it is not directly correlated with tissue damage. Long-term exercise training is an alert for athletes to modify or control the level of pain. There are different ways to control or decrease the pain (3), but those methods take time and athletes prefer to use fast methods.

It should be noted that, athletes normally use steroids and supplements to improve their performance and decrease the level of injuries, but those substances have also many side effects (4). They may also have an inhibitory effect on cellular regeneration and tissue healing (5).

Social pain

Pain includes sensory, emotional, cognitive and social dimensions that makes a negative experience for individuals (6, 7). Individuals experience different types of pain during their life such as physical or social pain (8) Social pain is defined as "the painful experience of actual or potential psychological distance from other people or social groups" (9). Social pain normally comes from the feeling of being human and described by symbolic meaning such as gestures or facial expressions (10). The negative feeling related to pain is related with physical pain (11) and social pain (12).

In fact, physical pain could get relieved earlier but the social pain has long term effect and athletes who face with social pain, will show unexpected psychological actions and social consequences. Studies have shown this relationship between physical pain and social pain, but the mechanism of this interaction is not determined yet. So, controlling and prevention of social pain, especially in athletes, who are under a huge pressure by society is very difficult (13).

Pain and law

In the United States, physicians are faced with two opposing dilemmas in the treatment of pain – the potential for drug abuse and diversion, and the possible under treatment of pain. There are different methods used by athletes to control and prevent pain, but most based on using steroids (14). Those drugs are expensive, but also costly in terms of addiction, overdose, death, and related criminal activities. Chronic pain carries significant economic, social, and health impact as well (15). National All Schedules Prescription Electronic Reporting (NASPER) Act of 2005, not only give some information regarding substance abuse but also help them to control it among athletes (16).

CONCLUSION

In this paper we found a relationship between physical and social pain in athletes. High levels of intensive exercise training and pressures made by competitions can lead to serious pain in athletes. They normally try to use substances to improve their pain, but those drugs have different types of side effects both for the athletes and also society. Injured athlete cannot control his/her emotions and will show unexpected action to other people if injured. There are some general guidelines in this regard, but there is a need to have a specific guidelines for the athletes and coaches to know how to prevent and how to control it. In addition, there is not a specific law for the athletes who did mistakes due to their physical and social pain.

REFERENCES

[1] Heidari J, Mierswa T, Kleinert J, Ott I, Levenig C, Hasenbring M, et al. Parameters of low back pain chronicity among athletes: associations with physical and mental stress. Phys Ther Sport 2016;21:31–7.

[2] Farahbakhsh F, Akbari-Fakhrabadi M, Shariat A, Cleland JA, Farahbakhsh F, Seif-Barghi T, et al. Neck pain and low back pain in relation to functional disability in different sport activities. J Exerc Rehabil 2018;14(3):509-12.

[3] Hosseini L, Shariat A, Ghaffari MS, Honarpishe R, Cleland JA. The effect of exercise therapy, dry needling, and nonfunctional electrical stimulation on radicular pain: a case report. J Exerc Rehabil 2018;14(5):864-73.

[4] Kargarfard M, Shariat A, Lam E, Shaw B, Shaw I, Shariat A. Prevalence and perceptions toward anabolic-androgenic steroid use amongst university students. Acta Medica Bulgarica. 2015;42(2).

[5] Davies L. Pain and the canine athlete: pain threshold, pain tolerance and drugs in competition. In: BSAVA Congress Proceedings 2020. BSAVA Library; 2020:296.

[6] Bonica JJ. The need of a taxonomy. Pain 1979;6:247–8.

[7] MacDonald G, Leary MR. Why does social exclusion hurt? The relationship between social and physical pain. Psychol Bull 2005;131(2):202.

[8] Eisenberger NI. Social pain and the brain: controversies, questions, and where to go from here. Annu Rev Psychol 2015;66:601–29.

[9] Eisenberger NI, Lieberman MD. Why it hurts to be left out: The neurocognitive overlap between physical and social pain. The social outcast: Ostracism, social exclusion, rejection, and bullying. 2005;109:130.

[10] Horing B, Sprenger C, Büchel C. The parietal operculum preferentially encodes heat pain and not salience. PLoS Biol 2019;17(8):e3000205.

[11] Xu X, Zuo X, Wang X, Han S. Do you feel my pain? Racial group membership modulates empathic neural responses. J Neurosci 2009;29(26):8525–9.

[12] Eisenberger NI. Broken hearts and broken bones: A neural perspective on the similarities between social and physical pain. Curr Direct Psychol Sci 2012;21(1):42–7.

[13] Zhang M, Zhang Y, Kong Y. Interaction between social pain and physical pain. Brain Sci Advanc 2019;5(4):265–73.

[14] Davis CS, Carr DH. The law and policy of opioids for pain management, addiction treatment, and overdose reversal. Ind Health L Rev 2017;14:1.

[15] Law LF, Sluka KA. How does physical activity modulate pain? Pain 2017;158(3):369.

[16] Manchikanti L, Whitfield E, Pallone F. Evolution of the National All Schedules Prescription Electronic Reporting Act (NASPER): A public law for balancing treatment of pain and drug abuse and diversion. Pain Physician 2005;8(4):335.

SECTION TWO: RESEARCH FINDINGS

In: Pain Management
Editors: J Merrick and M Morad
ISBN: 978-1-68507-493-7

Chapter 9

MUSCULOSKELETAL PAIN AND SONOGRAPHY FINDINGS

Dina Jalalvand*, MD and Pooneh Dehghan, MD
Department of Radiology, Shahid Beheshti University of Medical Sciences, Tehran, Iran

ABSTRACT

This chapter focus on recent sonography findings in musculoskeletal pains with the purpose of exploring the importance of these techniques in early detections. This work concludes the findings of previous studies about application of sonography for different types of musculoskeletal pains in neck, shoulder and lower back. To collect related papers, databases such as Google Scholar, Scopus, PubMed, and Cochrane were used and published English papers until November 2020 were considered. It was shown that, using sonography in early detection of musculoskeletal injuries and to make an accurate decision seems vital. So, as a practical message it is strongly suggested to attention to the

* ***Correspondence:*** Dina Jalalvand, MD, Mycobacteriology Research Center, National Research Institute of Tuberculosis and Lung Diseases (NRITLD), Shahid Beheshti University of Medical Sciences Tehran, Iran. Email: drdina.jalalvand@yahoo.com.

outcomes of sonography before any decision related to the individuals with musculoskeletal pains.

INTRODUCTION

Magnetic resonance imaging (MRI) was introduced in the 1980s and has revolutionized cross-sectional imaging of the musculoskeletal system and has ended up the foremost broadly utilized strategy for a wide assortment of pathologic conditions. The comprehensive depiction of osseous, and soft-tissue pathology given by MRI is unparalleled. For treatment choices, doctors and specialists depend intensely on the data given by MRI (1, 2).

Nevertheless, whereas MRI was picking up its authority, another musculoskeletal imaging method was introduced called sonography. Fast enhancements in innovation have made sonography an imperative complementary apparatus for musculoskeletal imaging, and there is presently an expansive body of writing reporting the adequacy of musculoskeletal sonography. With attention to the history of MRI and accurate presentation of reports, sonography stayed below rather than other radiology techniques, especially in developed countries (1, 3).

It should be noted that, sonography is easier to do and cheaper in cost, but the accuracy of MRI still seems higher. As sonography could be used as a fast technique in comparison with MRI, it could be useful for early detections of musculoskeletal injuries that would be the beginning for a musculoskeletal pain (4, 5).

With attention to this matter, this paper has tried to collect the practical information related to use of sonography in detection of musculoskeletal pain, based on the previous published papers.

MUSCULOSKELETAL PAIN

The pain related to musculoskeletal areas including the interaction among physical, social, psychological and environmental situations, so it is a practical framework to understand the biopsychosocial condition (6–8). Nowadays, muscusloskealtal pain is a worldwide problem and it could be directly related to the environment and society pressured made on individuals and it can affect the health system of people (9).

It is important to know that how the pain is created and when it is detected and how it is treated (10). Daily tasks of people and their job is also an important factor to occurrence of musculoskeletal pain. As it is shown in previous studies, long time sitting and longtime standing are the reasons for many types of musculoskeletal pains, especially in neck, shoulder and lower back area (11). Therefore, working situation is also an important item that should be noted by the physician in patients with pain.

Until now, there are different types of therapy suggested to prevent from or treatment of musculoskeletal pain. Using medicines is the most common type of therapy using by individuals to receive a fast result, but the side effects should be considered. In addition, those positive effects are temporary (12). Using modalities such as physiotherapy and occupational techniques are common among patients with pain (13). Prevention following regular exercise training is a recent way suggested by American College of Sports Medicine to prevent from occurrence of physical pain. It has no side effect and the cost is acceptable for everyone (14).

MUSCULOSKELETAL SONOGRAPHY

Sonography could be a symptomatic therapeutic method that employments high-frequency sound waves (ultrasound) to create energetic visual pictures of organs, tissues or blood stream interior the body. This sort of method is regularly alluded to as a sonogram or ultrasound exam (15).

With attention to the easy techniques of sonography and the acceptable cost in comparison with MRI, it is suggested by the experts. Scientists are trying to explore the benefits of sonography to improve the care of patients in different ways (16). Use of sonography, especially in rehabilitation settings such as physiotherapy and occupational therapy in monitoring the healing process and determine the changes over the time and providing feedback, is suggested (17). In spite of the fact that there is a call for expanded utilization of sonography by allied health suppliers, there is as of now restricted imaging substance inside proficient educational program, and numerous challenges exist in creating post-professional instruction and competency necessities. There is a lack of professional standard trainings and practice among countries to highlight the accuracy and available techniques of detection (18). In addition, using sonography in detection of physical injuries and pain needs to hours of experiences. At long last, to guarantee compelling usage, steady master mentoring is an imperative component of the post-professional prepare, something not promptly accessible for non-physicians (19).

CONCLUSION

Using sonography techniques is a useful and practical method to detect physical injuries and physical pain in early stages, but this need to enough experience and using standard techniques. MRI has some benefits in comparison with sonography, but it is expensive in cost and takes time to do. Still it is not clear if sonography could be useful for any type of physical pain and if there is any type of sonography that shows the points colorfully. More studies are needed to show the accurate abilities of doing sonography in early detection of physical pain in children, athletes and geriatrics.

REFERENCES

[1] Nazarian LN. The top 10 reasons musculoskeletal sonography is an important complementary or alternative technique to MRI. Am J Roentgenol 2008;190(6):1621–6.

[2] Kaplan PA, Matamoros Jr A, Anderson JC. Sonography of the musculoskeletal system. Am J Roentgenol 1990;155(2):237–45.

[3] Wooten A. Work-related musculoskeletal disorders in sonography. Radiol Technol 2019;90(3):215–24.

[4] Lee RKL, Griffith JF, Ng AWH, Tipoe GL, Chan AWH, Wong CWY, et al. Cross-sectional area of the median nerve at the wrist: Comparison of sonographic, MRI, and cadaveric measurements. J Clin Ultrasound 2019;47(3):122–7.

[5] Middleton WD, Payne WT, Teefey SA, Hildebolt CF, Rubin DA, Yamaguchi K. Sonography and MRI of the shoulder: comparison of patient satisfaction. Am J Roentgenol 2004;183(5):1449–52.

[6] Kittelson AJ, George SZ, Maluf KS, Stevens-Lapsley JE. Future directions in painful knee osteoarthritis: harnessing complexity in a heterogeneous population. Phys Ther 2014;94(3):422–32.

[7] Shariat A. Musculoskeletal disorders and their relationship with physical activities among office workers: A review. Malay J Public Health Med 2016;16(1):62–74.

[8] Shariat A, Tamrin SBM, Arumugam M, Danaee M, Ramasamy R. Office exercise training to reduce and prevent the occurrence of musculoskeletal disorders among office workers: a hypothesis. Malays J Med Sci 2016;23(4):54-9.

[9] Caneiro JP, Bunzli S, O'Sullivan P. Beliefs about the body and pain: the critical role in musculoskeletal pain management. Braz J Phys Ther 2020; S1413-3555(20)30407-X.

[10] Campbell P, Foster NE, Thomas E, Dunn KM. Prognostic indicators of low back pain in primary care: five-year prospective study. J Pain 2013;14(8):873–83.

[11] Shariat A, Alizadeh R, Moradi V, Afsharnia E, Hakakzadeh A, Ansari NN, et al. The impact of modified exercise and relaxation therapy on chronic lower back pain in office workers: a randomized clinical trial. J Exerc Rehabil 2019;15(5):703.

[12] Niculescu AB, Le-Niculescu H, Levey DF, Roseberry K, Soe KC, Rogers J, et al. Towards precision medicine for pain: Diagnostic biomarkers and repurposed drugs. Mol Psychiatry 2019;24(4):501–22.

[13] Calner T, Isaksson G, Michaelson P. Physiotherapy treatment experiences of persons with persistent musculoskeletal pain: a qualitative study. Physiother Theory Pract 2019; 27:1–10.

[14] Medicine AC of S. ACSM's exercise is medicine: a clinician's guide to exercise prescription. Philadelphia, PA: Lippincott Williams Wilkins, 2009.

[15] Sanders RC, Winter TC. Clinical sonography: a practical guide. Philadelphia, PA: Lippincott Williams Wilkins, 2007.

[16] Akkaya N, Ulash AM, Özçakar L. Use of musculoskeletal ultrasound in clinical studies in physiatry: the "stethoscope" is also becoming the "pen. J Rehabil Med 2013;45(7):701–2.

[17] Roll SC, Asai C, Tsai J. Clinical utilization of musculoskeletal sonography involving non-physician rehabilitation providers: A scoping review. Eur J Phys Rehabil Med 2016;52(2):253-9.

[18] Gray JM, Frank G, Roll SC. Integrating musculoskeletal sonography into rehabilitation: therapists' experiences with training and implementation. OTJR (Thorofare N J) 2017;37(1):40–9.

[19] Cole B, Twibill K, Lam P, Hackett L, Murrell GAC. Not all ultrasounds are created equal: general sonography versus musculoskeletal sonography in the detection of rotator cuff tears. Shoulder Elbow 2016;8(4):250–7.

In: Pain Management
Editors: J Merrick and M Morad
ISBN: 978-1-68507-493-7

Chapter 10

THE BRIEF PAIN INVENTORY (BPI), HEBREW VERSION: A PSYCHOMETRIC VALIDATION

Motti Ratmansky[1], MD, Pesach Shvartzman[2,3], MD, Tamar Freud[2], PhD, Tali Samson[2,3], PhD and Amir Haim[1,*], MD, PhD

[1]Pain Rehabilitation Unit, Loewenstein Rehabilitation Hospital, Raanana, Israel
Sackler Faculty of Medicine, Tel Aviv University, Tel Aviv, Israel
[2]Family Medicine Department and Siaal Research Center for Family Medicine and Primary Care, Faculty of Health Sciences, Ben-Gurion University of the Negev, Beer Sheva, Israel
[3]Pain and Palliative Care Unit, Faculty of Health Sciences, Ben-Gurion University of the Negev, Beer Sheva, Israel

[*] Corresponding Author's Email: amirhaim@gmail.com.

ABSTRACT

The Brief Pain Inventory (BPI) is a simple tool for the assessment of pain and its impact, widely used in clinical and research pain medicine. It has been translated and validated in many languages. Despite its widespread use in Israel, it has undergone linguistic validation only. We devised the current study to complete a psychometric validation of the Hebrew version of the BPI. Methods: The study included 163 patients from two pain clinics. Patients were asked to complete the questionnaire twice, once before the beginning of a routine visit and again at its conclusion (an interval of about 30 minutes). Confirmatory factor analysis (CFA), explanatory factor analysis (EFA), and internal consistency reliability analyses were conducted. Results: Of the 163 patients, 53.4% were females, and the mean age was 57.65 ± 16.45 years. The most common diagnosis was low back pain (58.9%). CFA confirmed the 2-factor structure of the BPI (pain interference and pain severity). In the EFA, 11 BPI items were loaded onto two factors. The rotated solution of the two factors accounted for 63.29% of the variance. We found a high degree of correlation between test and retest results for each item separately and for each of the two subscales: pain severity ($r = 0.877$, $p < 0.001$) and pain interference ($r = 0.855$, $p < 0.001$). Conclusion: The Hebrew version of the BPI is a useful and reliable tool to assess pain in Hebrew speaking non-cancer pain patients.

ABBREVIATIONS

BPI	Brief Pain Inventory
CFA	Confirmatory factor analysis
EFA	explanatory factor analysis
CFI	comparative fit index
NFI	Normed Fit Index
NNFI, also known as TLI	Non-Normed Fit Index
RMSEA	Root mean squared error approximation
KMO	Kaiser–Meyer–Olkin
EORTC QLQC-30	European Organization for Research and Treatment of Cancer quality of life 30-item core questionnaire

INTRODUCTION

The Brief Pain Inventory (BPI) is a questionnaire that is simple and easy to use for the assessment of pain. This tool, which was originally designed to measure the severity and impact of pain on daily function in cancer patients (1), has also been used effectively in patients with pain from other causes, such as AIDS-related pain (2) and pain due to sickle cell disease. We found this questionnaire to be useful for the assessment of chronic pain in non-cancer patients in an ambulatory pain clinic. Its use enables pain practitioners to monitor their patients' status from visit to visit and evaluate the effect of treatment. Since it difficult to evaluate pain objectively based on the report of pain sufferers or caregivers, a validated measure of the severity and impact of pain on daily function is of immense importance.

In Israel the BPI has been popularized and utilized for clinical and research in the field of pain medicine, including in cancer patients (3,4), Parkinson's disease (5), the general population (6), hemodialysis patients (7) and soldiers on active duty (8). Despite its widespread use in Israel, the instrument has undergone linguistic validation only, so the psychometric characteristics of the Hebrew version have not been assessed to date. The aim of the present study was to conduct a psychometric validation of the Hebrew version of the BPI.

OUR STUDY

The study was approved by the ethics committees of Meir Medical Center in Kfar Saba, Israel and the Loewenstein Hospital in Raanana, Israel.

The BPI is a self-administered instrument that evaluates two parameters of pain. The first is severity, assessed by four items that describe pain: [a] the worst pain over the past 24 hours, [b] the weakest pain over the past 24 hours, [c] the average pain, and [d] the severity of the current pain at the time of the survey.

The second estimates the degree of impact that the pain has on daily function, assessed by seven questions relating to the effect of pain on: [a] general activity, [b] mood, [c] ambulation, [d] routine work, [e] relationships with other people, [f] sleep, and [g] life pleasure.

The BPI was developed in England and evaluated on cancer patients (1). Its psychometric characteristics have been assessed in different populations and in different languages, including Italian (9), German (10), Hindi (11), Greek (12), Norwegian (13), Russian (14), Thai (15), Polish (16), Brazilian Portuguese (17) and Spanish (18).

Settings

The study was conducted in two pain clinics in Israel, the Pain Rehabilitation Clinic at Loewenstein Hospital in Raanana and the Pain Relief Clinic of the Southern District of the Clalit Healthcare Services in Beer Sheva. The study was approved by the Helsinki Committees of the Meir Medical Center in Kfar Saba and the Loewenstein Hospital in Raanana, Israel.

Sample size

A rule of thumb for the calculation of sample size for factor analyses is a ratio of 10:1 between the number of items in the questionnaire and the number of respondents (19). A smaller ratio increases the risk of finding a strong fit between the model and the sample even when one does not actually exist. In the present study, we chose a ratio of 15:1 for each item in the instrument, with the aim of keeping to the rule of thumb and reducing the risk of a mistake. Since the BPI contains 11 items, we included 164 participants from the two clinics.

Inclusion criteria

Patients with chronic pain. Ambulatory patients coming to the pain clinic for their first visit, or for a follow-up visit that did not involve invasive therapy (injections). Patients 18 years of age and above. Patients who speak Hebrew at a level that enables them to understand and discuss items in the questionnaire (reading ability was not required).

Exclusion criteria

Patients diagnosed with an active malignant disease.

Hebrew translation

The Hebrew version of the questionnaire was provided by the developers of the original questionnaire.

Data collection

The questionnaires were completed at the time of a routine visit to one of the study clinics. Patients were asked to complete the questionnaire twice, once at the beginning of the visit and again at its conclusion (an interval of about 30 minutes). At the first administration, the respondents were asked to complete the socio-demographic items and the physicians were asked to record the principal medical diagnosis.

Data analyses

The data were processed using the SPSS and AMOS software package (Version 22). In the first stage, univariate analyses were performed to describe the socio-demographic characteristics of the respondents. Mean and standard deviations were calculated for each BPI item.

Confirmatory factor analysis (CFA), explanatory factor analysis (EFA), and internal consistency reliability analyses were conducted on the questionnaires at the first administration. This timing was chosen to minimize bias stemming from familiarity with the questionnaire and the potential effect of the visit with a pain specialist on the degree of pain (exacerbation or alleviation of the subjective pain level).

Confirmatory factor analysis

The structure of the Hebrew version of the BPI questionnaire was assessed by CFA to test the degree of fit between the Hebrew version and the original questionnaire. The indices that were recorded for this assessment were Normed $\chi 2$ ($\chi 2$/df), comparative fit index (CFI), Normed Fit Index (NFI(, Non-Normed Fit Index (NNFI, also known as TLI) and root mean squared error approximation (RMSEA) (20). Hu and Bentler (21) suggested that, for continuous data, the cutoff points should be RMSEA < 0.06, CFI > 0.95, TLI > 0.95, and Normed $\chi 2$ < 2 5.

Exploratory factor analysis

In accordance with the results, an EFA was conducted with principal axis and direct oblimin rotation. The analysis included items whose loading value for a factor was moderate or above, at = 30. The number of factors was determined by the number of factors with an eigenvalue above 1.

Reliability assessment

Internal consistency reliability - to assess the reliability of the BPI, coefficient alphas were computed for interference and severity scales.

Correlation coefficients between each item and the total scale were calculated and the effect of deleting items on the Cronbach alpha values was examined. Test-retest reliability - Spearman's correlation coefficient was used to calculate the correlation of BPI scores between time 1 (pre-visit) and time 2 (post-visit) at the level of individual items.

FINDINGS

The study included 163 patients who visited one of the two study pain clinics. Of these, 53.4% were females, mean age was 57.65 ± 16.45 years, 63.1% were born in Israel, 71.7% were married, 48.1% had 9-12 years of education, almost 95% were Jewish, and 47.9% were secular. The most common diagnoses were low back pain (58.9%) and neuropathic pain (15.6%) (see Table 1).

Table 1. Socio-demographic characteristics of the study population (N = 163)

		N	%	Total
Gender	Male	76	46.6%	163
	Female	87	53.4%	
Age	Mean ± STD	57.65 ± 16.45		158
	Range	24-88		(mis = 6)
Country of birth	Israel	99	63.1%	157
	Abroad	58	36.9%	(mis = 6)
Years in Israel	Mean ± STD	51.81 ± 15.49		58
	Range	11-78		
Marital status	Single	13	8.2%	159 (mis = 4)
	Divorced	12	7.5%	
	Widowed	16	10.1%	
	Married	114	71.7%	
	Separated	4	2.5%	

Table 1. (Continued)

		N	%	Total
Education (years)	0-4	3	1.9%	156 (mis = 7)
	5-8	16	10.3%	
	9-12	75	48.1%	
	13-15	35	22.4%	
	16+	27	17.3%	
Employment	Salaried employee	45	28.8%	156 (mis = 7)
	Partially salaried employee	14	9.0%	
	Self-employed	10	6.4%	
	Retired	40	25.6%	
	Housewife	7	4.5%	
	Unemployed	10	6.4%	
	Receives an allowance	25	16.0%	
	Other	5	3.2%	
Religion	Jew	149	94.9%	157 (mis = 6)
	Muslim	8	5.1%	
Are you?	Traditional	48	33.8%	142 (mis = 21)
	Religious	23	16.2%	
	Orthodox	3	2.1%	
	Secular	68	47.9%	
Diagnosis (more than one is possible)	Low back pain	83	58.9%	141 (mis = 22)
	Neuropathic pain	22	15.6%	
	Fibromyalgia	10	7.1%	
	Cervical pain	10	7.1%	
	Shoulder pain	9	6.4%	
	Myofascial pain	6	4.3%	
	Osteoarthritis	6	4.3%	
	Joint pain	5	3.5%	
	Hip pain	5	3.5%	
	CRPS	4	2.8%	
	Limb pain	3	2.1%	
	Chest symptoms	2	1.4%	
	Headache	1	0.7%	
	Other	15	10.6%	

Confirmatory factor analysis

The CFA was used to determine the degree of fit between identified factors from the Hebrew version with known factors from the English version, i.e., pain interference and pain severity. The BPI model with two dimensions showed a good fit to data: $\chi2 = 89.15$, df = 43, $\chi2/df = 2.073$, CFI = 0.949, NFI = 0.908, TLI = 0.921 and RMSEA = 0.081 (CI 90% 0.057-0.105). Since the RMSEA index had a moderate fit only, we conducted an EFA to enhance our understanding of the questionnaire structure.

Exploratory factor analysis

Using an EFA based on the principal axis factoring method with oblimin rotation and a factor coefficient of 0.35 or greater, 11 BPI items were loaded onto two factors (see Table 2). The first factor (interference) included 7 items that accounted for 53.97% of the total variance in the matrix with an eigenvalue of 5.937. The second factor (pain) included four items that accounted for 9.32% of the common variance with an eigenvalue of 1.033.

Table 2. Exploratory factor analysis

BPI Items	Factor	
	1	2
Worst pain		0.660
Least pain		0.707
Average pain		0.581
Current pain		0.892
General activity	0.686	
Mood	0.765	
Ambulation	0.543	
Work	0.734	
Relationships	0.749	
Sleep	0.509	
Pleasure	0.855	
Eigen	5.937	1.033
% of Variance	53.97	9.32

The rotated solution of the two factors accounted for 63.29% of the variance. The Kaiser–Meyer–Olkin (KMO) measure of sampling adequacy value was 0.91 and the Bartlett's test of sphericity was highly significant ($\chi2 = 771.81$, df = 55, $p < 0.000$).

Internal consistency reliability

To assess the reliability of the BPI, we calculated the coefficient alpha separately for the pain severity scale (four pain severity items) and the pain interference scale (seven interference items). Table 3 shows a summary of the BPI scores and the coefficient alpha results.

Table 3. Summary of Brief Pain Inventory (BPI) scores by item and internal consistency in the study population

BPI Items	Item Statistics		Subscale	Correlation with total	Alpha with item deleted
	Mean	SD			
Worst pain	7.8	1.9	Severity (Cronbach's Alpha = 0.835)	0.619	0.816
Least pain	4.5	2.9		0.694	0.787
Average pain	6.5	1.9		0.700	0.788
Current pain	5.9	2.8		0.718	0.770
General activity	7.1	2.4	Interference (Cronbach's Alpha = 0.888)	0.744	0.866
Mood	6.3	2.9		0.727	0.865
Ambulation	5.7	3.4		0.582	0.885
Work	7.2	2.6		0.739	0.866
Relationships	4.5	3.5		0.748	0.863
Sleep	6.4	3.2		0.589	0.883
Pleasure	6.8	2.7		0.705	0.869

The mean pain severity levels ranged from 4.5 ± 2.9 to 7.8 ± 1.9. The mean pain interference levels ranged from 4.5 to 7.1 across the seven items. The internal consistency of the two subscales was high (above the accepted limit of 0.70), with Cronbach's alpha = 0.835 in the pain severity subscale and Cronbach's alpha = 0.888 in the pain interference subscale. As can be seen in Table 2, the Cronbach's alpha suggests that each of the items contributes similarly to the underlying construct that it is intended to measure, even if an item is deleted.

Test-retest reliability

Table 4 demonstrates the results of test-retest reliability between time 1 (pre-visit) and time 2 (post-visit) BPI assessments at the individual item level. We found a high degree of correlation between test and retest results for each item separately and for each of the two subscales: pain severity ($r = 0.877$, $p < 0.001$) and pain interference ($r = 0.855$, $p < 0.001$).

Table 4. Test-retest reliability of Brief Pain Inventory (BPI) questionnaires before and after visiting the pain physician

Item	Test	Retest	Correlation Coefficient	P value
Worst pain	7.8	7.7	0.807	<0.0001
Least pain	4.5	4.9	0.790	<0.0001
Average pain	6.5	6.5	0.699	<0.0001
Current pain	5.9	6.0	0.807	<0.0001
Pain severity subscale	**6.2**	**6.3**	**0.877**	**<0.0001**
General activity	7.1	6.9	0.671	<0.0001
Mood	6.3	6.0	0.744	<0.0001
Ambulation	5.7	5.7	0.806	<0.0001
Work	7.2	6.6	0.793	<0.0001
Relationships	4.5	4.5	0.814	<0.0001
Sleep	6.4	6.1	0.875	<0.0001
Pleasure	6.8	6.1	0.677	<0.0001
Pain interference subscale	**6.3**	**6.0**	**0.855**	**<0.0001**

CONCLUSION AND DISCUSSION

The present study evaluated the psychometric properties of the BPI Hebrew version in patients with non-cancer pain. The results of the study support the originally hypothesized two-factor structure, comprised of pain severity and pain interference (1), that was also found in other studies (9,10,12,13,15-18,21). In contrast, other BPI validation studies have identified three factors: pain severity, activity interference and affective interference (11,22-25).

The CFA in our study provided evidence for the validity of the two-factor model that was also demonstrated in the validation of the Brazilian BPI (17). The results of two BPI confirmatory factor analyses in patients with painful bone metastases (25) in HIV/AIDS and on cancer patients (22) provided evidence for the validity of the three-factor model.

Cronbach's alpha coefficients for both severity and interference items were high (Cronbach's alpha = 0.835 and Cronbach's alpha = 0.888, respectively). These values exceed 0.7, a typical standard for acceptable scale stability. Other BPI validation studies also identified high Cronbach's alpha coefficients values for both factors (9,10,12-18).

We examined the reliability of the BPI test, not only on the basis of correlation coefficients but also on test-retest stability. As in the study by Radbruch et al. (10), the patients in our study completed the BPI before and after consultation in the pain clinic, with at least a 30-minute interval between test and retest. We found high correlation rates between test and retest in both the pain severity and pain interference subscales (r = 0.877 and r = 0.855, respectively). The correlation coefficients for pain severity and interference did not change between the test and the retest (Cronbach's alpha = 0.835 and 0.888 for the test and 0.885 and 0.912 for the retest). In another study performed on cancer pain patients, the test-retest process was performed at four points in time: before treatment and on the 7th, 8th, and 14th days of pain therapy. The authors concluded that the BPI is sensitive to changes in both pain severity and pain interference resulting from therapy (16).

The main limitation of our study was that we did not test whether the Hebrew version of the BPI actually measures the pain construct. Other BPI validation studies have validated BPI results against the Short-Form 36 Health Survey (SF36) (10,13,14) or the European Organization for Research and Treatment of Cancer quality of life 30-item core questionnaire (EORTC QLQC-30)(16,17,23). Based on previous studies, we assumed that the Hebrew version does measure the pain construct, so we decided to focus on psychometric validation of the Hebrew version.

In conclusion, based on the results of the present study, we can safely state that the Hebrew version of the BPI is a useful and reliable tool to assess pain in Hebrew-speaking non-cancer pain patients.

ACKNOWLEDGEMENTS

No conflict of interest in any author.

REFERENCES

[1] Cleeland CS, Ryan KM. Pain assessment: Global use of the Brief Pain Inventory. Ann Acad Med Singapore 1994;23:129-38.

[2] Breitbart W, McDonald MV, Rosenfeld B, et al. Pain in ambulatory AIDS patients. I: Pain characteristics and medical correlates. Pain 1996;68:315-21.

[3] Shvartzman P, Friger M, Shani A, Barak F, Cohen Y, Singer Y. Pain control in ambulatory cancer patients--can we do better? J Pain Symptom Manage 2003;26(2):716-22.

[4] Cohen MZ, Musgrave CF, Munsell MF, Mendoza TR, Gips M. The cancer pain experience of Israeli and American patients 65 years and older. J Pain Symptom Manage 2005;30(3):254-63.

[5] Djaldetti R, Yust-Katz S, Kolianov V, Melamed E, Dabby R. The effect of duloxetine on primary pain symptoms in Parkinson disease. Clin Neuropharmacol 2007;30(4):201-5.

[6] Neville A, Peleg R, Singer Y, Sherf M, Shvartzman P. Chronic pain: A population-based study. Isr Med Assoc J 2008;10(10):676-80.

[7] Golan E, Haggiag I, Os P, Bernheim J. Calcium, parathyroid hormone, and vitamin D: major determinants of chronic pain in hemodialysis patients. Clin J Am Soc Nephrol 2009;4:1374-80.

[8] Eilat-Tsanani S, Tabenkin H, Lavie I, Castel OC, Merom L. The effect of low back pain on work absenteeism among soldiers on active service. Spine (Phila Pa 1976) 2010;35(19):E995-9.

[9] Caraceni A, Mendoza TR, Mencaglia E, Baratella C, Edwards K, Forjaz MJ, et al. A validation study of an Italian version of the Brief Pain Inventory (Breve Questionario per la Valutazione del Dolore). Pain 1996;65(1):87-92.

[10] Radbruch L, Loick G, Kiencke P, Lindena G, Sabatowski R, Grond S, et al. Validation of the German version of the Brief Pain Inventory. J Pain Symptom Manage 1999;18(3):180-7.

[11] Saxena A, Mendoza T, Cleeland CS. The assessment of cancer pain in north India: the validation of the Hindi Brief Pain Inventory--BPI-H. J Pain Symptom Manage 1999;17:27-41.

[12] Mystakidou K, Mendoza T, Tsilika E, Befon S, Parpa E, Bellos G, et al. Greek brief pain inventory: validation and utility in cancer pain. Oncology 2001;60(1):35-42.

[13] Gjeilo KH, Stenseth R, Wahba A, Lydersen S, Klepstad P. Validation of the brief pain inventory in patients six months after cardiac surgery. J Pain Symptom Manage 2007;34(6):648-56.

[14] Kalyadina SA, Ionova TI, Ivanova MO, Uspenskaya OS, Kishtovich AV, Mendoza TR, et al. Russian Brief Pain Inventory: validation and application in cancer pain. J Pain Symptom Manage 2008;35(1):95-102.

[15] Chaudakshetrin P. Validation of the Thai Version of Brief Pain Inventory (BPI-T) in cancer patients. J Med Assoc Thai 2009;92:34-40.

[16] Leppert W, Majkowicz M. Polish brief pain inventory for pain assessment and monitoring of pain treatment in patients with cancer. J Palliat Med 2010;13:663-8.

[17] Ferreira KA, Teixeira MJ, Mendonza TR, Cleeland CS. Validation of brief pain inventory to Brazilian patients with pain. Support Care Cancer 2011;19:505-11.

[18] de Andres Ares J, Prado LMC, Verdecho MAC, Villanueva LP, Hoyos MDV, Herdman M, et al. Validation of the Short Form of the Brief Pain Inventory (BPI-SF) in Spanish patients with non-cancer-related pain. Pain Pract 2015;15(7):643-53.

[19] Costello AB, Osborne JW. Best practices in exploratory factor analysis: Four recommendations for getting the most from your analysis. Pract Assessment 2005;10:1-9.

[20] McDonald RP, Ho MH. Principles and practice in reporting structural equation analyses. Psychol Methods 2002;7:64-82.

[21] Hu L, Bentler PM. Cutoff criteria for fit indexes in covariance structure analysis: Conventional criteria versus new alternatives. Struct Equ Modeling 1999;6:1-55.

[22] Atkinson TM, Rosenfeld BD, Sit L, Mendoza TR, Fruscione M, Lavene D, et al. Using confirmatory factor analysis to evaluate construct validity of the Brief Pain Inventory (BPI). J Pain Symptom Manage 2011;41(3):558-65.

[23] Klepstad P, Loge JH, Borchgrevink PC, Mendoza TR, Cleeland CS, Kaasa S. The Norwegian brief pain inventory questionnaire: translation and validation in cancer pain patients. J Pain Symptom Manage 2002;24(5):517-25.

[24] Mendoza T, Mayne T, Rublee D, Cleeland C. Reliability and validity of a modified Brief Pain Inventory short form in patients with osteoarthritis. Eur J Pain 2006;10:353-61.

[25] Wu JS, Beaton D, Smith PM, Hagen NA. Patterns of pain and interference in patients with painful bone metastases: a brief pain inventory validation study. J Pain Symptom Manage 2010;39:230-40.

In: Pain Management
Editors: J Merrick and M Morad
ISBN: 978-1-68507-493-7

Chapter 11

Chronic Non-Malignant Pain with Central and Primary Hypogonadism

Arun Aggarwal*, MBBS, FRACP, FAFRM (RACP), FFPMANCZA, PhD and Monica Ling, MBBS, FAFRM (RACP)

RPAH Pain Management Centre, Camperdown,
Sydney and Department of Rehabilitation Medicine,
Prince of Wales Hospital, Randwick, New South Wales, Australia

Abstract

Chronic non-malignant pain is a common condition affecting up to 22% of the general population. There have been a number of studies investigating the role of the endocrine system in chronic pain. We performed a nine month prospective, cross-sectional analysis of all male patients with chronic non-malignant pain who were referred to a tertiary multi-disciplinary pain clinic to investigate whether chronic non-malignant pain caused biochemical hypogonadism, regardless of the

* ***Correspondence:*** A/Professor Arun Aggarwal, RPAH Pain Management Centre, RPAH, Camperdown, Sydney, NSW, Australia 2139. Email: arun.a@sydney.edu.au.

impact of opioids. We had a sample size of 66 male patients, with an average age of 51 years (age range 15-86 years). Their average duration of pain was 8.1 years. 41 males were receiving oral opioids (including oxycodone, morphine, methadone and combination analgesia containing codeine and tramadol) and 25 males were on non-opioid treatment (including simple analgesics, anti-inflammatories and adjuvant medications such as anti-convulsants and anti-depressants). Results showed that 35 males had no evidence of hypogonadism, 17 males had biochemical evidence of central (hypogonadotrophic) hypogonadism due to suppression of the hypothalamic-pituitary-gonadal axis and 14 males had evidence of primary hypogonadism due to testicular disease (congenital, excessive alcohol and increasing age). We conclude that hypogonadism is a common complication of chronic non-malignant pain, irrespective of opioid use. Both central (hypogonadotrophic) and primary hypogonadism occurs in this condition and is strongly correlated with the age of the patient and duration of pain. This is the first study to demonstrate an association between biochemical hypogonadism and chronic non-malignant pain, itself.

INTRODUCTION

Chronic non-malignant pain is a common condition affecting up to 22% of the general population. It has detrimental effects on physical and emotional functioning, quality of life and ability to work. Complete relief of chronic pain occurs infrequently, and is likely related to the limited knowledge regarding the underlying pathophysiology (1). The current understanding is that chronic pain is a dynamic phenomenon involving changes in the peripheral and central nervous system in response to disease, injury or loss of function (2).

There have been a number of studies investigating the role of the endocrine system in chronic pain. All of these studies have assessed the impact of opioids on the endocrine system, rather than the effect of chronic pain itself.

It is known that the hypothalamic-pituitary-adrenal axis is altered in females with fibromyalgia, but no studies have addressed the importance of the hypothalamic-pituitary-gonadal axis (3). Of this axis, testosterone is the principal androgen. Production occurs 95% in the testes and 5% in the adrenals, and is regulated by the hypothalamus and pituitary through a negative feedback system. 98% is bound to sex-hormone-binding globulin and albumin, and only 2% is in the free, biologically active form (4). The two main effects of testosterone are virilization resulting in development of the male secondary characteristics, and anabolic effects on muscle, bone, energy, mood and libido (5).

The causes of hypogonadism are classified as either primary due to testicular impairment from age, viral orchitis, trauma, radiation, drugs, excessive alcohol, autoimmunity, granulomatous disease and systemic disease; or secondary due to central hypothalamic-pituitary suppression from pituitary tumours, or suppression from opioids and stressors such as hypoglycaemia, hypotension, trauma, infection, exercise or chronic illness (6).

It has been shown that the gonadal axis is centrally suppressed in chronic pain treated with intrathecal opioids (7). Our hypothesis is that chronic pain itself, irrespective of whether treatment is opioid or non-opioid based, may lead to hypogonadism in males.

OUR STUDY

A prospective, cross-sectional analysis was carried out on all male patients with chronic non-malignant pain referred to a multi-disciplinary pain clinic over a nine month period. Subjects were excluded if they were already on androgen replacement therapy or corticosteroids.

Data was obtained via interviews on: age of patient, duration, site and cause of the chronic pain, and medications. Blood samples were collected and assays of: total and free serum testosterone, sex-hormone-binding globulin, free-androgen index, lutenising and follicular-stimulating hormones. All testosterone, LH and FSH levels were performed in the same laboratory to allow standardisation of hormone levels. This reduces the variability between laboratories.

The biochemical results were grouped according to whether they were hypogonadic (low total or free testosterone or low free-androgen index) or normal. Those with hypogonadism were further subdivided into a central hypogonadotrophic group (normal or low LH/FSH) and a primary hypogonadic group (high LH/FSH).

FINDINGS

66 male patients with chronic non-malignant pain were studied. It was not necessary for any subjects to be excluded based on our exclusion criteria. Of these 66 patients, 35 had normal biochemistry, 17 had biochemical evidence of central hypogonadism, and 14 had primary hypogonadism (see Figure 1). The average age of the 66 male subjects was 51.1 years (range 15-86 years).

Table 1. Results of all three groups

	Normal	Central hypogonadic	Primary hypogonadic
Number	35	17	14
Average Age (yrs)	45.1 (15-72)	56.9 (34-80)	59.2 (39-86)
Ave Duration of Pain (yrs)	6.2 (0.5-22)	10.8 ().5-30)	9.9 (0.16-25)
Mean LH (1-10)	4.9	4.5	17.1
Mean FSH (1-8.5)	5.3 (1.1-11.2)	6.1 (2.6-15.3)	30.8 (11-92.8)
Free Testosterone (170-510)	263.8 (178-586)	145.4 (56-227)	130.3 (31-321)
Oral Opioids	54%	76%	64%
Weaker Opioids	75%	50%	80%
Strong Opioids	25%	50%	20%
Non-Opioids	46%	24%	36%

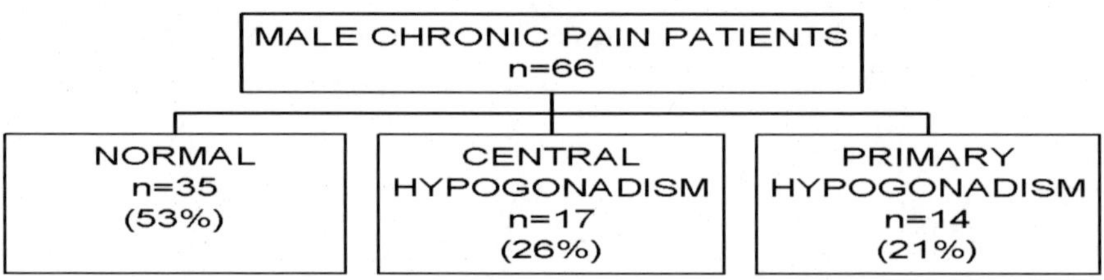

Figure 1. Flowchart of biochemical results.

Duration of Pain

The average duration of pain was 8.1 years (range 0.5-30 years). In patients with pain lasting less than 10 years, they were 1.5 times more likely to be normal (n=21) than hypogonadic (n=14). It was the converse for patients with pain lasting more than 10 years, as they were 1.5 times more likely to be hypogonadic (n=15) than normal (n=10) (see Figure 2). The mean LH level (normal 1-10) was 7.4 (range 0.7-55.9), and the mean FSH level (normal 1-8.5) was 10.9 (range 1.1-92.8). The average free testosterone level (normal 170-510) was 204 (range 31-586).

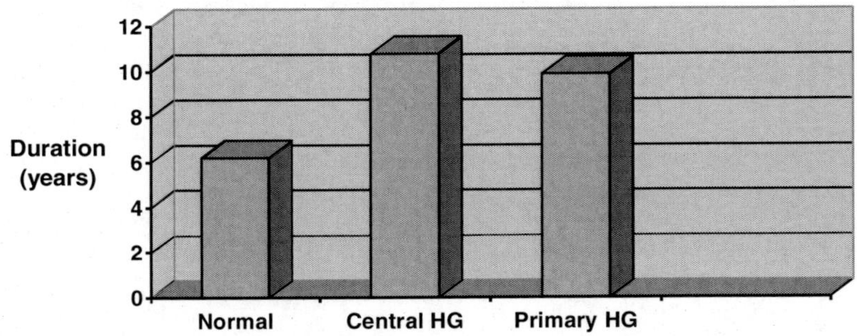

Figure 2. Comparison of duration of pain.

Site of pain

The most common site of pain was the lumbar region (n=36), followed by the leg (n=22), arm (n=17), other sites (n=14) such as the abdomen, ribs and generalised body pain, cervical spine (n=9) and head (n=7).

Cause of pain

The cause of pain was work related (n=13), trauma (n=15), degenerative disease (n=12), unknown (n=14), or other causes (n=12) such as surgery, congenital scoliosis or herpes zoster infection.

Medications

62% of patients were receiving oral opioid medication (n=41), of which two-thirds (n=27) were on weak opioids, i.e., low doses of paracetamol and codeine and tramadol, and one-third (n=14) were on stronger opioids such as oxycodone, morphine and methadone.

38% of patients were receiving non-opioid medications which included, simple analgesia, anti-epileptic medications, NSAID's, COX-II inhibitors, tricyclic antidepressants, SSRI's, and others such as cannabis and alcohol.

Normal group (n=35)

The average age of the 35 male subjects was younger at 45.1 years (range 15-72 years). The average duration of pain was lower at 6.2 years (range 0.5-22 years). The mean LH level was 4.9 (range 0.9-10), and the mean FSH level was 5.3 (range 1.1-11.2). The average free testosterone level was 263.8 (range 178-586). The site and cause of pain was similar to that of the total group. 54% of patients were receiving oral opioid medications (n=19), of which 75% were on weaker opioids (n=14) and 25% were on stronger opioids (n=5). 46% were on non-opioid medications which were distributed evenly in the total group.

Central hypogonadic group (n=17)

The average age of the 17 male subjects was older, at 56.9 years (range 34-80 years). The average duration of pain was longer, at 10.8 years (range 0.5-30 years). The mean LH level was 4.5 (range 0.7-9.6), and the mean FSH level was 6.1 (range 2.6-15.3). The average free testosterone level was low, at 145.4 (range 56-227). The site and cause of pain was similar to that of the total group. A higher proportion of patients (76%) were receiving oral opioid medications (n=13), of which 50% were on weaker opioids (n=6) and 50% were on stronger opioids (n=7). 24% of patients were on non-opioid medications which were distributed evenly in the total group.

Primary hypogonadic group (n=14)

The average age of the 14 male subjects was older, at 59.2 years (range 39-86 years). The average duration of pain was longer, at 9.9 years (range 0.16-25 years). The mean LH level was high, 17.1 (range 6.9-55.9), as was the mean FSH level at 30.8 (range 11-92.8). The average free testosterone level was subnormal, at 130.3 (range 31-321). The site and cause of pain was similar to that of the total group. 64% of patients were receiving oral opioid medications (n=9), of which 80% were on weaker opioids (n=7) and 20% were on stronger opioids (n=2). 36% were on non-opioid medications which were again distributed evenly in the total group.

Although strong opioids (oxycodone, morphine and methadone) were more commonly associated with central hypogonadism (n=7), strong opioids could also lead to no biochemical abnormalities (n=5). There was statistical significant correlation between the groups (see Figure 3).

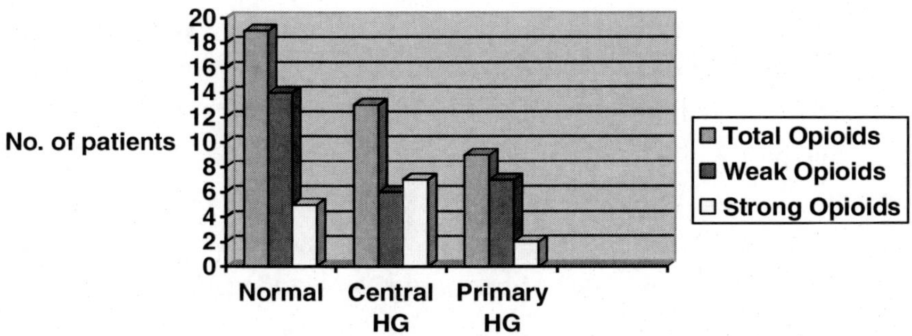

Figure 3. Comparison of patients receiving oral opioids.

Conclusion

Our results demonstrate that hypogonadism, both central and primary, is associated with chronic non-malignant pain. In this study we found hypogonadism in 47% of our male study group. Of these hypogonadic patients, approximately half had a central form of hypogonadism and the other half had primary hypogonadism.

From our results, it appears that the association between chronic pain and hypogonadism is distinct from the effect of opioid therapy. Therefore, other factors must be involved in the relationship between these patients and their hypogonadism, such as age and the duration of pain.

It is unknown from our study, whether chronic pain causes hypogonadism, as there have been no previous studies in the literature which have documented this relationship. Chronic stress however is known to cause hypogonadism in animals, via suppression of the hypothalamic-pituitary-testicular axis in animals (8, 9). It has been postulated that this is due to a modification in LHRH secretion, rather than a reduction in pituitary responsiveness to LHRH. Studies have been performed on females with fibromyalgia, which have shown the definite suppression of the hypothalamic-pituitary-adrenal axis (10) Interestingly, it has been previously hypothesised that the hypothalamic-pituitary-adrenal axis may modulate the hypothalamic-pituitary-gonadal axis via CRH causing inhibition of GnRH secretion (11) If this hypothesis is valid, then this would also be a plausible explanation for the hypogonadism seen in chronic pain.

Several large studies have shown that hypogonadism is associated with depression, independent of age, weight change and physical activity (12). Hypogonadism has also been linked with anxiety, irritability, insomnia, weakness, reduced libido, impotence, poor memory and reduced muscle and bone mass (13).

From our results, hypogonadism appears to be much more strongly correlated with the age of the patient and duration of chronic pain, rather than oral opioid medication. The age of the patient seems to be the most important predictor for hypogonadism. In younger patients aged less than

50 years, they were three times more likely to be normal (n=23) than hypogonadic (n=8). Older patients aged more than 50 years were 2 times more likely to be hypogonadic (n=23) than normal (n=12).

This is not unexpected, as more knowledge has been increasingly discovered regarding a "male menopause" or "andropause." Although it is a concept that is still debated as it is not as inevitable as the female menopause, it has been proven that plasma testosterone concentrations do fall in middle aged and elderly men, up to 50% compared with young men (14). The mechanism whereby this occurs, is thought to be via both a decline in Leydig cell mass in the testicles, and a dysfunction in hypothalamic-pituitary homeostatic control. This would explain why our hypogonadic patients had a mixed central and primary testicular distribution.

The duration of the chronic pain is also an important factor, as the longer the duration of chronic pain, the more likely to have hypogonadism. In patients with pain lasting less than 10 years, they were 1.5 times more likely to be normal (n=21) than hypogonadic (n=14). It was the converse for patients with pain lasting more than 10 years, as they were 1.5 times more likely to be hypogonadic (n=15) than normal (n=10), see Figure 1.

There are numerous studies regarding the impact of opioids on the endocrine system (15). There have been previous studies on endogenous opioids, heroin and methadone addicts and chronic pain patients on intrathecal opioids which have all demonstrated an association with central hypogonadism (16-19). This has been thought to be due to occupation of the opiate receptors in the hypothalamus leading to central hypothalamic suppression of GnRH secretion (20). The fact that our hypogonadic patients displayed an almost equivalent amount of central as well as primary hypogonadism, suggests that opioids alone are unable to account for the association with chronic pain.

Our results indicated that although strong opioids (oxycodone, morphine and methadone) were more commonly associated with central hypogonadism (n=7), strong opioids could also lead to no biochemical abnormalities (n=5). This association was not statistically significant.

In the interpretation of our results, we are aware of a few study limitations. Although the sample size was 66, and much larger than those used in previous studies, a larger population would improve the reliability of our findings. As this was designed to be a prospective, cross-sectional analysis, it was unable to be determined whether the association between hypogonadism and chronic pain was due to cause or effect. We are aware that the breakdown between strong and weak opioids is a somewhat artificial categorisation, but in the weak opioid group low doses of paracetamol and codeine and tramadol were used and in the stronger opioids group, high doses of oxycodone, morphine and methadone were used. Some of the non-opioid medications can also have a minor effect on gonad function, but these patients were not excluded from the study.

Regardless of the aetiology of the hypogonadism which may in fact be multifactorial, the question is raised as to whether or not such hypogonadism should be treated with androgen supplementation. Again, there are no previous studies to address this direct question.

In studies of chronic pain patients on intrathecal morphine with evidence of both central and primary hypogonadism, testosterone supplementation resulted in improved libido, sexual function, mood, muscle mass and strength, as well as improved rehabilitation outcomes in terms of Functional Independence Measure and grip strength in ill older hypogonadic men (21, 22). However, any effects on the chronic pain itself were not reported. Thus, although androgen supplementation should seriously be considered in hypogonadic chronic pain patients, it should be implemented with caution as long term studies on its efficacy and safety are lacking (23).

This is the first study to consider that chronic pain may be an independent factor in hypogonadism, regardless of the impact of the use of oral or intrathecal opioids, as central and primary hypogonadism occurs in chronic non-malignant pain. It is most strongly associated with age of the patient and duration of the chronic pain, rather than opioid intake.

ACKNOWLEDGMENTS

There were no funding sources required for this study. The authors declare that they have no conflict of interest. Informed consent was obtained from each individual participant involved in this study. This study was conducted in accordance with the 1964 Declaration of Helsinki and its subsequent amendments.

REFERENCES

[1] Ashburn MA, Staats PS. Management of chronic pain. Lancet 1999;353: 1865-9.

[2] Nurmikko TJ, Nash TP. Control of chronic pain. BMJ 1998;317:1438-41.

[3] Clauw DJ, Chrousos GP. Chronic pain and fatigue syndromes: overlapping clinical and neuroendocrine features and potential pathogenic mechanisms. Neuroimmunomodulation 1997;4:134-53.

[4] Basaria S, Dobs AS. Hypogonadism and androgen replacement therapy in elderly men. Am J Med 2001;110(7) 563-72.

[5] Winters SJ. Androgens:endocrine physiology and pharmacology. NIDA Res Monogr 1990;102:113-30.

[6] Griffin JE, Wilson JD. Disorders of the testes and male reproductive tract. In: Wilson JD, Foster DW, eds. Williams textbook of endocrinology, 7th Ed. Philadelphia, PA: WB Saunders, 1985:259-311.

[7] Finch PM, Roberts LJ. Hypogonadism in patients treated with intrathecal morphine. Clin J Pain 2000;16:251-4.

[8] Knol BW. Stress and the endocrine hypothalamus-pituitary-testis system: a review. Vet Q 1991;13(2):104-14.

[9] Lopez-Calderon, Ariznavarreta C. Stress induced changes in testis function. J Steroid Biochem Mol Biol 1991;40(1-3):473-9.

[10] Adler GK, Kinsley BT. Reduced hypothalamic-pituitary and sympathoadrenal responses to hypoglycaemia in women with fibromyalgia syndrome. Am J Med 1999;106(5):534-43.

[11] Crofford LJ. Neuroendocrine abnormalities in fibromyalgia and related disorders. Am J Med Sci 1998;315(6):359-66.

[12] Barrett-Connor E, Von Muhlen DG. Bioavailable testosterone and depressed mood in older men: the rancho bernado study. J Clin Endocrinol Metab 1999; 84:573-7.

[13] Sternbach H. Age-Associated testosterone decline in men: Clinical issues for psychiatry. Am J Psychiatry 1998;155(10):1310-8.

[14] Klee GG, Heser, DW. Techniques to measure testosterone in the elderly. Mayo Clin Proc 2000;75(Suppl):s19-25.

[15] Katz N, Mazer NA. The impact of opioids on the endocrine systems. Clin J Pain 2009;25(2):170-5.

[16] Azizi F, Vagenakis A. Decreased serum testosterone concentration in male heroin and methadone addicts. Steroids 1973;22:467-72.

[17] Pelosi MA, Sama JC. Galactorrhea-amenorrhea syndrome associated with heroin addiction. Am J Obstet Gynecol 1974:118:966-70.

[18] Cicero TJ, Bell RD. Function of the male sex organs in heroin and methadone users. N Engl J Med 1975;292:882-7.

[19] Wang C, Chan V. The effect of heroin addiction on pituitary-testicular function. Clin Endocrinol (Oxf) 1978;9:455-61.

[20] Cicero TJ. Effects of exogenous and endogenous opiates on the hypothalamic-pituitary-gonadal axis in the male. Fed Proc 1980;39(8):2551-4.

[21] Wang C, Swerdloff RS. Transdermal testosterone gel improves sexual function, mood, muscle strength, and body composition parameters in hypogonadal men. J Clin Endocrinol Metab 2000;85:2839-53.

[22] Bakhshi V, Eilliott M. Testosterone improves rehabilitation outcomes in ill older men. JAGS 2000;48:550-3.

[23] Daniel HW. Hypogonadism in men consuming sustained-action oral opioids. J Pain 2002;3(5):377-84.

In: Pain Management
Editors: J Merrick and M Morad
ISBN: 978-1-68507-493-7

Chapter 12

OLDER ADULTS WITH CHRONIC LOW BACK PAIN: FUNCTIONAL DISABILITY AND QUALITY OF LIFE

Orapin Laosee[1,*], PhD, Netchanok Sritoomma[2], PhD, Phanida Wamontree[3], PhD, Cheerawit Rattanapan[1], PhD, Wichian Tansuwanond[4,5], MD and Chitr Sitthi-Amorn[6,7], MD, PhD

[1]ASEAN Institute for Health Development, Mahidol University, Nakorn Pathom, Thailand
[2]PhD Nursing Management Program and College of Nursing, Christian University of Thailand, Nakorn Pathom, Thailand
[3]School of Integrative Medicine, Mae Fah Luang University, Chiang Rai, Thailand
[4]Damnoen Saduak Hospital, Ratchaburi, Thailand

* ***Correspondence:*** Orapin Laosee, ASEAN Institute for Health Development, Mahidol University, 999 Salaya, Phudthamonthon, Nakorn Pathom, Thailand. Email: Orapin.lao@mahidol.edu.

[5]Health Promotion Center Region 5, Department of Health, Ministry of Public Health, Nonthaburi, Thailand
[6]Saint Louis College, Bangkok
[7]Faculty of Medicine, Chulalongkorn University, Bangkok, Thailand

ABSTRACT

To determine the association of functional disability and quality of life (QOL) among older adults with chronic low back pain. Methods: Participants were adults aged 60 years or older diagnosed with chronic low back pain in out-patient departments. Subjects were asked to assess their pain level, functional disability and quality of life. A multiple logistic regression was carried out to identify the independent variables associated with QOL. Results: A total of 406 participants were recruited with an average age of 68.9 year (SD 7.2), the majority of whom were female (70.9%). Most participants reported having a poor QOL (83.7%). Multivariate analysis revealed that being female (aOR 1.84, 95% CI 1.03 - 3.30), at an age of 70 years and older (aOR 2.18, 95% CI 1.16 - 4.08), in severe pain (aOR 2.19, 95% CI 1.17 - 4.10), and had problems with social contacts (aOR 3.35, 95% CI 1.88 - 5.96) were more likely to report a poor level of QOL. Conclusions: Lower quality of life is reported in chronic low back pain patients. Social life related factors need to be further investigated to improve QOL among older people.

INTRODUCTION

Low back pain (LBP) is a worldwide public health problem with a lifetime prevalence of 84% (1). Previous studies have found the incidence of LBP is highest in the third decade of life, and overall prevalence increases with age (1-3). It was estimated that the number of years lived with disability caused by LBP increased by 54% between 1990 and 2015, with the majority of the increase being seen in ageing populations in low- and middle-income countries (4). With the rapid growth of the elderly population worldwide, LBP has become increasingly important both medically and socioeconomically. A systematic analysis of the Global Burden of Disease study for 2016 reported that among 328 diseases, LBP was the fifth leading cause of years lived with disability (5). Moreover, prevalence and burden increases with age, with a peak at 80 years of age (6). LBP is a very commonly reported musculoskeletal condition among older patients visiting primary care facilities (7). Chronic LBP can negatively impact patient quality of life (QOL) as a result of pain, with impaired mobility, decreased social activity and changes in mood (1, 8-10).

QOL is one of the key indicators in assessing an individual's health and well-being. As defined by the World Health Organization (11), QOL is the perception of an individual's position in life in the context of their culture and value systems, and is influenced by their goals, expectations, experiences, standards, beliefs and concerns. There are four domains related to QOL; physical health, psychological health, social relationships and environment. Limits on physical function (8, 12-18), increased psychological frailty (19), and reduced social engagement and low social capital (20) were significantly associated with QOL in previous research studies. These studies also showed that the elderly with LBP were at risk of becoming frail in relation to higher levels of functional limitations, psychological difficulties and social restrictions, leading to poor QOL (21, 22).

Studies of the impact of LBP on health-related QOL in old age reported that among sufferers, pain was chronic, occurred on most or every day and limited daily activities (9, 15). Because of limited research in this area, the purpose of this study was to ascertain how functional disability related to QOL among elderly patients with chronic LBP.

OUR STUDY

This was a cross-sectional study in four community hospitals, representing four different regions of Thailand. The hospital directors were contacted to obtain permission prior to data collection. Four research assistants in each hospital were trained to ensure competency in collecting the study measurements. Simple random sampling was employed to recruit 100-105 subjects per a hospital. A total of 410 patients aged 60 years and older who had been diagnosed with chronic LBP by a physician from May-August 2017 was enrolled. Chronic LBP was defined as suffering the symptom of LBP for at least 12 weeks prior to recruitment in the study.

MEASUREMENT

QOL was assessed using the World Health Organization Quality of Life instrument (WHOQOL-BREF THAI) (Department of Mental Health, Thailand). WHOQOL-BREF THAI consisted of two types of questions, perceived objective and self-reporting subjective. There were 26 items measuring four broad domains, physical health (seven items), psychological (six items), social relationships (three items), and environment (eight items). Respondents scored the items of QOL for the previous two weeks on a 5-point Likert response scale (range 1-5). QOL was categorized into two groups, poor and good, according to the standard score. Higher scores indicated higher QOL and a better perception as to their health. Pain density was assessed with the Visual Analog Scale, categorizing it as mild to moderate (score 1-6), and severe (> 6). The Oswestry Low Back Pain Disability Questionnaire, which consisted of 10 questions, was used to identify pain intensity and its effect on personal care, lifting, walking, sitting, standing, sleeping, social contact and travelling. The respondents reported which activities they could engage in without extra pain as "no problem;" however, if there was extra pain then it was classified as a "problem."

Procedure

Ethical clearance was obtained from the institutional review board of Mahidol University. Data was collected in out-patient departments of each hospital. The research assistants systematically approached the participants and invited them to participate. After their consent, the subjects were interviewed. The interview took approximately 20 minutes to complete for each respondent.

Statistical analysis

Descriptive statistics were employed to determine central distribution and frequency of the study variables. Binary logistic regression was used to determine the factors associated with QOL. Variables with a p-value < 0.25 in binary logistic regression were included in the multivariable model. A p-value < 0.05 was considered statistically significant. Crude odds ratios (OR) and adjusted ORs (aOR) were reported for associations between variables and QOL levels, with 95% confidence intervals (95% CI).

FINDINGS

Mean age of respondents was 68.9 years (standard deviation, SD 7.2), and 70.9% were female. Over three-quarters (77.1%) had completed primary education, and approximately half (47.0%) were still working. The majority considered themselves in severe pain (46.3%), and 83.7% had a poor perception of their QOL (see Table 1).

The top three functional disabilities due to LBP were problems of lifting (91.4%), standing (87.8%), and sitting (84.7%; see Figure 1).

Table 2 shows the results of bivariate regression analyses of characteristics and functional disability and QOL. The analyses revealed that gender, age group, marital status, disability level, pain level, ability to walk, sleeping and social contact were statistical significantly associated with QOL.

Table 1. Descriptive characteristics of the respondents (n = 406)

Characteristics		**n (%)**
Sex	Female	288 (70.9)
Age (years)	60 - 69	248 (61.1)
	70 - 79	117 (28.8)
	80+	41 (10.1)
	Mean age 68.9, SD 7.2	
Education level	No school	34 (8.4)
	Primary	313 (77.1)
	Higher than primary	59 (14.5)
Current work	Not working/retired	215 (53.0)
	Agriculture	110 (27.1)
	Employee	81 (20.0)
Marital status	Married	262 (64.5)
	Single*	144 (35.5)
Exercise	No	230 (56.7)
	Yes	176 (43.3)
Pain level	Mild to moderate	218 (53.7)
	Severe	188 (46.3)
QOL level	Poor	340 (83.7)
	Good	66 (16.3)

*Single represents those that are single, divorced, or widowed.

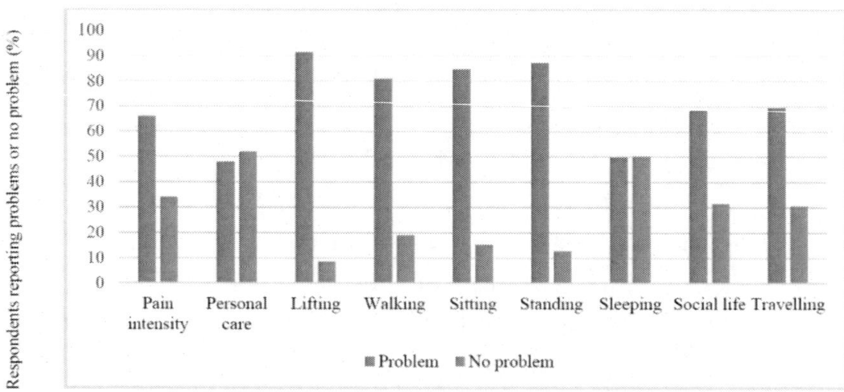

Figure 1. Proportion of respondents who report problems/no problems with regard to functional disability.

Table 2. Bivariate analysis of QOL level and independent variables

		Quality of life level			
		Good	**Poor**	**OR (95%CI)**	**p-value**
		n (%)	**n (%)**		
Characteristics of subjects					
Sex	Female	37 (12.8)	251 (87.2)	2.21 (1.28 - 3.80)	0.004
	Male	29 (24.6)	89 (75.4)	1	
Age (years)	60 - 69	49 (19.8)	199 (80.2)	1	
	70+	17 (10.8)	141 (79.7)	2.04 (1.12 - 3.69)	0.018
Education level	Primary and lower	54 (15.6)	293 (84.4)	1.38 (0.69 - 2.78)	0.360
	Higher than primary	12 (20.3)	47 (79.7)	1	
Current work	Not working/retried	33 (15.3)	182 (84.7)	1.15 (0.68 - 1.95)	0.599
	Working	33 (17.3)	158 (82.7)	1	
Marital status	Married	51 (19.5)	211 (80.5)	1	
	Single*	15 (10.4)	129 (89.6)	2.07 (1.12 - 3.84)	0.020
Exercise	No	34 (14.8)	196 (85.2)	1.28 (0.75 - 2.17)	0.358
	Yes	32 (18.2)	144 (81.8)	1	
Disability level	Up to moderate	63 (20.7)	241 (79.3)	1	
	Severe +	3 (2.9)	99 (97.1)	8.62 (2.64 - 28.11)	< 0.001
Pain level	Mild	49 (22.5)	169 (77.9)	1	
	Severe	17 (9.0)	171 (91.0)	2.91 (1.61 - 5.26)	< 0.001
Functional disability					
Pain intensity	No problem	20 (14.5)	118 (85.5)	1	
	Problem	46 (17.2)	222 (82.8)	0.81 (0.46 - 1.44)	0.490
Personal care	No problem	40 (19.0)	171 (81.0)	1	
	Problem	26 (13.3)	169 (86.7)	1.52 (0.88 - 2.60)	0.127
Lifting	No problem	9 (25.7)	26 (74.3)(7)	1	
	Problem	57 (15.4)	314 (84.6)	1.90 (0.84 - 4.28)	0.118
Walking	No problem	21 (27.3)	56 (72.7)	1	
	Problem	45 (13.7)	284 (86.3)	2.36 (1.30 - 4.28)	0.004
Sitting	No problem	13 (21.0)	49 (79.0)	1	
	Problem	53 (15.4)	291 (84.6)	1.45 (0.74 - 2.86)	0.277
Standing	No problem	12 (23.1)	40 (76.9)	1	
	Problem	54 (15.3)	300 (84.7)	1.66 (0.82 - 3.38)	0.157
Sleeping	No problem	48 (23.5)	156 (76.5)	1	
	Problem	18 (8.9)	184 (91.1)	3.14 (1.75 - 5.63)	< 0.001
Social contact	No problem	40 (31.3)	88 (68.8)	1	
	Problem	26 (9.4)	252 (90.6)	4.40 (2.54-3.95)	< 0.001
Travelling	No problem	25 (20.2)	99 (79.8)	1	
	Problem	41 (14.5)	241 (85.5)	1.48 (0.85 - 2.57)	0.159

QOL, quality of life; OR, odds ratio, CI, confidence intervals. *Single represents those that are single, divorced, or widowed.

Multivariate analyses identified that those that were female (aOR 1.84, 95% CI 1.03 - 3.30), at an age of 70 years and older (aOR 2.18, 95% CI 1.16 - 4.08), in severe pain (aOR 2.19, 95% CI 1.17 - 4.10), and had problems with social contacts (aOR 3.35, 95% CI 1.88 - 5.96) were more likely to have a poor QOL (see Table 3).

Table 3. Multivariate analysis of QOL of the respondents

Variables		Adjusted Odds Ratio (95% CI)	p-value
Sex	Male	1	
	Female	1.84 (1.03 - 3.30)	0.040
Age	60 - 69	1	
	70+	2.18 (1.16 - 4.08)	0.014
Pain level	Mild to moderate	1	
	Severe	2.19 (1.17 - 4.10)	0.014
Social contact	No problem	1	
	Problem	3.35 (1.88 - 5.96)	< 0.001

DISCUSSION

This study reported that the majority (83.7%) of elderly with LBP reported poor levels of QOL. LPB was shown to be related to QOL, limiting their ability in all activities, especially lifting, walking, standing, social life and travelling. In general, it is difficult to compare results across QOL studies with the elderly due to different measurements used and different perceptions with regard to life conditions, culture, goals, standards, norms and value systems.

A study of Japanese adults with chronic LBP showed that a higher somatic symptom burden was significantly associated with a lower health-related QOL (23). Our study also found functional disabilities, such as walking, sleeping, and social contact, were associated with QOL. Previous studies have suggested that other somatic symptom burden could lead to a worse LBP outcome and lower QOL as a consequence (22, 24-26). A research study was conducted on the effect of LBP on health-related QOL in a large sample of elderly Swiss living in the community (15). It showed that pain for the participants was chronic, occurred most or every day and induced activity limitations in over half of the sample. In addition, individuals reporting pain every day, severe pain and more than three years since their last episode without pain, lost 10 points on the scale of health-related QOL (15).

A high percentage of respondents in our study had problems with common daily life activities, such as standing (84.7%), sitting (84.7%), and walking (81.0%), which were related to lower QOL. Similar to our study, regression analysis on community dwelling older adults aged 65 years and older showed that individual suffering from LBP had significantly more problems, such as pain/discomfort, mobility, usual activities, anxiety and self-care (8). In addition, elderly at risk became frail in terms of their higher level of functional limitation, psychological difficulties and social restriction.

The current study highlighted that social life played an important role in QOL. Social networks were also one of the key factors related to QOL of adults living in South Korea (27). This study indicated that social networks could support health-related QOL, and possibly health-promoting behavior. A cross-sectional survey of 825 people aged 60 years and older in rural counties of China reported that there was a significant association between low social capital and poorer health related to QOL. Social life is an important element in relation to QOL in Asian countries, and could similarly be reflected in many cultures. Asia consisted of many ancient cultures with diverse religions, beliefs and life philosophies. A study of social participation, willingness to participate and QOL among older adults in rural area of China was conducted. The findings revealed that subjects who participated in social activities were more likely to have high scores of health-related QOL (28). Those who reported high social contact and support utilization were inclined to engage in social participation. The initiation of social participation programs to increase social interaction for older adult with LBP should be considered, and could be integrated in existing Thai cultural activities.

This study had a number of limitations. These included it being a cross sectional study which assessed functional disability and perception of QOL at only a point in time. Some participants might not have been totally honest in their perception, due to the discomfort in sharing personal information. Thus, reports by participants should be understood as being limited to their own perceptions of the issues.

CONCLUSION

This study was consistent with previous reports on older adults with chronic LBP who seek treatment in community hospitals. Individuals declared that pain affect their physical abilities, including walking, standing, sitting and social life, leading to a poor QOL. Special consideration could be taken of the elderly who were female, ≥ 70 years of age, had severe pain, and who had less social contact. The results highlight the importance of radiating chronic LBP, low mobility, and social life when considering risks of loss in QOL.

ACKNOWLEDGMENTS

The research study was funded by Thailand Research Fund Grant No. MRG6080282. We thank all older adults who participated in this study. The authors declare that they have no conflict of interest.

REFERENCES

[1] Balagué F, Mannion AF, Pellisé F, Cedraschi C. Non-specific low back pain. Lancet 2012;379(9814):482-91.

[2] Hoy D, Brooks P, Blyth F, Buchbinder R. The epidemiology of low back pain. Best Pract Res Clin Rheumatol 2010;24(6):769-81.

[3] Hoy D, March L, Brooks P, Woolf A, Blyth F, Vos T, et al. Measuring the global burden of low back pain. Best Pract Res Clin Rheumatol 2010;24(2):155-65.

[4] Hartvigsen J, Hancock MJ, Kongsted A, Louw Q, Ferreira ML, Genevay S, et al. What low back pain is and why we need to pay attention. Lancet 2018;391(10137):2356-67.

[5] Vos T, Abajobir AA, Abbafati C, Abbas KM, Abate KH, Abd-Allah F, et al. Global, regional, and national incidence, prevalence, and years lived with disability for 328 diseases and injuries for 195 countries, 1990-2016: A systematic analysis for the Global Burden of Disease Study 2016. Lancet 2017;390(10100):1211-59.

[6] Hoy D, March L, Brooks P, Blyth F, Woolf A, Bain C, et al. The global burden of low back pain: Estimates from the Global Burden of Disease 2010 study. Ann Rheum Dis 2014;73(6):968-74.

[7] Wettstein M, Eich W, Bieber C, Tesarz J. Pain intensity, disability, and quality of life in patients with chronic low back pain: Does age matter? Pain Med 2019;20(3):464-75.

[8] Cedraschi C, Luthy C, Allaz AF, Herrmann FR, Ludwig C. Low back pain and health-related quality of life in community-dwelling older adults. Eur Spine J 2016;25(9):2822-32.

[9] Kim W, Jin YS, Lee CS, Hwang CJ, Lee SY, Chung SG, et al. Relationship between the type and amount of physical activity and low back pain in koreans aged 50 years and older. PM R 2014;6(10):893-9.

[10] Duncan RP, Van Dillen LR, Garbutt JM, Earhart GM, Perlmutter JS. Low back pain - related disability in Parkinson disease: Impact on functional mobility, physical activity, and quality of life. Phys Ther 2019;99(10):1346-53.

[11] World Health Organization. The World Health Organization Quality of Life Instrument (WHOQOL). Geneva: World Health Organization, 2018.

[12] Murata S, Doi T, Sawa R, Saito T, Nakamura R, Isa T, et al. Association between joint stiffness and health-related quality of life in community-dwelling older adults. Arch Gerontol Geriatr 2017;73:234-9.

[13] Puciato D, Borysiuk Z, Rozpara M. Quality of life and physical activity in an older working-age population. Clin Interv Aging 2017;12:1627-34.

[14] Johansson L, Sundh D, Nilsson M, Mellström D, Lorentzon M. Vertebral fractures and their association with health-related quality of life, back pain and physical function in older women. Osteoporos Int 2018;29(1):89-99.

[15] Ludwig C, Luthy C, Allaz AF, Herrmann FR, Cedraschi C. The impact of low back pain on health-related quality of life in old age: results from a survey of a large sample of Swiss elders living in the community. Eur Spine J 2017;27(5):1154-65.

[16] Quah JHM, Wang P, Ng RRG, Luo N, Tan NC. Health-related quality of life of older Asian patients with multimorbidity in primary care in a developed nation. Geriatr Gerontol Int 2017;17(10):1429-37.

[17] Storey S, Gray TF, Bryant AL. Comorbidity, Physical Function, and Quality of Life in Older Adults with Acute Myeloid Leukemia. Curr Geriatr Rep 2017;6(4):247-54.

[18] Morisaki N. Relationship between swallowing functions and health-related quality of life among community-dwelling dependent older individuals. Jpn J Nurs Sci 2017;14(4):353-63.

[19] Van Der Vorst A, Zijlstra GAR, De Witte N, Vogel RGM, Schols JMGA, Kempen GIJM, et al. Explaining discrepancies in self-reported quality of life in frail older people: A mixed-methods study. BMC Geriatr 2017;17(1):251.

[20] Zhong Y, Schön P, Burström B, Burström K. Association between social capital and health-related quality of life among left behind and not left behind older people in rural China. BMC Geriatr 2017;17(1):287.

[21] Gobbens RJJ, van Assen MALM. Associations between multidimensional frailty and quality of life among Dutch older people. Arch Gerontol Geriatr 2017;73:69-76.

[22] Kim W, Jin YS, Lee CS, Bin SI, Lee SY, Choi KH. Influence of Knee Pain and Low Back Pain on the Quality of Life in Adults Older Than 50 Years of Age. PM R 2015;7(9):955-61.

[23] Fujii T, Oka H, Katsuhira J, Tonosu J, Kasahara S, Tanaka S, et al. Association between somatic symptom burden and health-related quality of life in people with chronic low back pain. PLoS One 2018;13(2):e0193208.

[24] Matsudaira K, Konishi H, Miyoshi K, Isomura T, Inuzuka K. Potential risk factors of persistent low back pain developing from mild low back pain in urban Japanese workers. PLoS One 2014;9(4):e93924.

[25] Nickel R, Egle UT, Rompe J, Eysel P, Hoffmann SO. Somatisation predicts the outcome of treatment in patients with low back pain. J Bone Joint Surg Series B 2002;84(2):189-95.

[26] Ailliet L, Rubinstein SM, Knol D, van Tulder MW, de Vet HCW. Somatization is associated with worse outcome in a chiropractic patient population with neck pain and low back pain. Man Ther 2016;21:170-6.

[27] Hong M, De Gagne JC, Shin H. Social networks, health promoting-behavior, and health-related quality of life in older Korean adults. Nurs Health Sci 2018;20(1):79-88.

[28] He Q, Cui Y, Liang L, Zhong Q, Li J, Li Y, et al. Social participation, willingness and quality of life: A population-based study among older adults in rural areas of China. Geriatr Gerontol Int 2017;17(10):1593-602.

In: Pain Management
Editors: J Merrick and M Morad
ISBN: 978-1-68507-493-7

Chapter 13

CALMARE® THERAPY AND TRANSCUTANEOUS ELECTRICAL NERVE STIMULATION IN RANDOMIZED PERIPHERAL NEUROPATHY SUBJECTS WITH RESTING STATE FMRI MONITORING

Ty A Bodily, BS, MS, Logan Edvalson, BS, Jordan B Peacock, BS, Zack M Bradshaw, BS, Carson Hart, BS, Cameron Ernst, BS, Samuel Biggs, BS and David D Busath*, BA, MS, MD

Department of Physiology and Developmental Biology
and Center for Neuroscience, Brigham Young University,
Provo, Utah, United States of America

* ***Correspondence:*** David D. Busath, MD, Retired Professor of Physiology and Biophysics, Department of Physiology and Developmental Biology, LSB 4005, College of Life Sciences, Brigham Young University, Provo, UT 84602, United States.
Email: david.busath@gmail.com.

ABSTRACT

Clinical reports of Calmare® protocol efficacy suggest enhanced durability compared to TENS and the possibility of changes in resting fMRI connectivity. The objective was to compare peripheral neuropathy pain relief and resting fMRI changes with Calmare and TENS treatments. Randomized double-blind trials were performed in August 2015 and between August 2016 and November 2017, with 18 and 20 human peripheral neuropathy subjects, respectively. The initial trial examined effects of a single session while the latter trial examined the effects of a course of ten treatment sessions on consecutive weekdays. fMRI scans were examined for changes in blood flow correlations and connectivity. Subjective pain scores were similarly reduced by both Calmare and TENS treatments in both studies. In the ten-session study the relief was prolonged, again similarly for both groups. The pain area relieved, which may be a more important metric than residual pain score, was reduced significantly more in the Calmare group than in the TENS group in *post hoc* analysis. After treatment, resting fMRI showed an increase in global efficiency and in correlation of activity between left hippocampus and right amygdala for both treatment modalities. Treatment with Calmare or TENS yields prolonged pain reduction and correlates with reproducible fMRI changes.

INTRODUCTION

Multiple studies have shown that transcutaneous electrical nerve stimulation (TENS) effectively reduces hyperalgesia and allodynia in neuropathy patients (1, 2) as well as subjects with spinal cord injury (3, 4). Scrambler therapy, using the Calmare® device (Calmare Therapeutics Inc, Fairfield, CT, USA) and referred to here as Calmare treatment, is a transcutaneous electrical treatment that has also demonstrated significant ability to alleviate neuropathic pain according to one review (5). Subsequently, reduction of chronic post-mastectomy pain (6) and chemotherapy-induced peripheral neuropathy (CIPN) (7-9), and neuromyelitis optica (10) were also reported with Calmare. However, to our knowledge, no reports of efficacy comparison between Calmare and TENS nor of fMRI correlates of pain reduction have been published.

We evaluated whether Calmare efficacy was greater or more durable than TENS in subjects with peripheral neuropathy. Randomized prospective double-blind studies of one-session and ten-session treatment regimens were conducted with resting state fMRI before and after treatment periods and upon later return. Subjects scored their burning superficial pain, which, together with paresthesia and numbness, is a common symptom in peripheral neuropathy (11, 12).

The neural network that processes acute pain includes regions of the insular, secondary somatosensory, and anterior cingulate cortices, as well as thalamus, and hypothalamus (13). There is less consensus on brain regions involved with chronic pain. One metastudy found that low back pain, post-herpetic neuralgia, and osteo-arthritic knee pain have different fMRI signatures in spontaneous and evoked pain paradigms (14). Similarly, gray-matter volumes change differentially in chronic back pain, complex regional pain syndrome, and knee osteoarthritis (15). Nevertheless, fMRI with chronic pain often shows aberrant connectivity involving the anterior cingulate gyrus, insula, medial prefrontal cortex, precuneus, amygdala, striatum, hippocampus, thalamus, tegmentum, nucleus accumbens, and periaqueductal gray (16-22). Placebo and sham effects are well-known to affect perception of acute (23) and chronic (24) pain and central mechanisms mediating placebo effects have been hypothesized (25-27). Here, we take advantage of analgesia from Calmare and TENS to examine changes in resting state network activation for idiopathic peripheral neuropathy subjects.

Our Study

Subject selection

Subject anonymity was protected by the protocol reviewed and approved by the Brigham Young University Internal Review Board, Protocol F15130 and registered as NCT04242797 at clinicaltrials.gov. Eighteen subjects for the one-session study and twenty for the ten-session study were chosen from a pool of interested candidates with chronic pain conditions and gave written informed consent (see Figure 1).

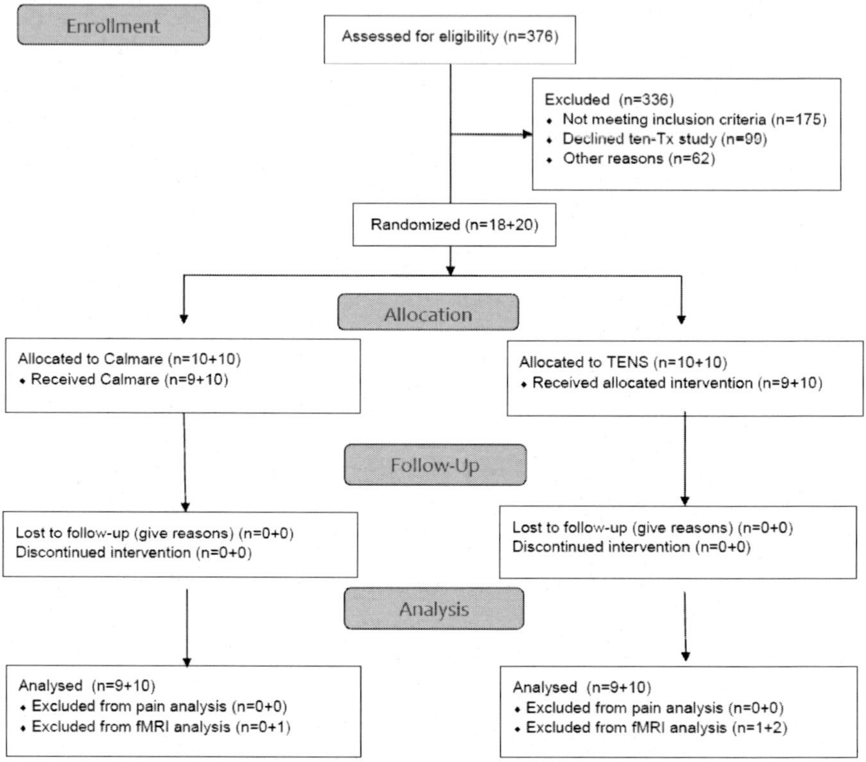

Figure 1. CONSORT 2010 Flow Diagram: Randomized clinical trial selection for both the one-treatment and the ten-treatment study. The number of subjects in the two studies are designated as one-session count + ten-session count where appropriate. Of 376 subjects that volunteered for study in response to advertisements, the first 18 meeting the study criteria were selected for the preliminary one-treatment study, nine randomly assigned to each group (Calmare vs. TENS). Seven of those assigned to the TENS group opted to return three weeks later for unmasked Calmare treatment as a crossover group. The following year, all of the original volunteers that were qualified and had current contact information, except for the eighteen in the one-treatment study, were called back and invited to participate in the ten-treatment study. The twenty that were qualified and willing were identified and randomly assigned to each group (Calmare vs. TENS). Exclusions from the fMRI analysis were due to data loss.

Sample size for the ten-session study was based on treatment efficacy observations from the one-session study. Inclusion criteria included a diagnosis by a medical doctor of peripheral neuropathy, preferably idiopathic, a pain rating higher than 4 (on a scale of 1-10), and minimal medication history subject to exclusion criteria (see Table S1). Candidates taking pregabalin, topiramate, gabapentin or tramadol were asked to consult with their physician prior to discontinuing the medications two weeks before the study to reduce medication variability and because they are suspected to inhibit Calmare efficacy. They were not excluded from the trial if they were unable, such that a few subjects were included who took these medications up to a few days before beginning the study and, in one case, during the study. Subjects were assigned to groups by the blind-manager for each study using a random number generator and an algorithm to assign similar gender blocks for each treatment block, and assignments were well-matched between groups for their gender, age, diagnosis, and drug history (see Tables S1 and S2). Pain was most frequently described as burning and sharp, starting in the feet, and moving proximally as the disease progressed. This manuscript adheres to Consort 2010 guidelines.

Study protocols

In the one-session study, the subjects received an initial fMRI, the double-blind treatment, and a second fMRI on day one, then returned for a third fMRI on day two. The nine subjects in the TENS group were invited two weeks later for a non-blind Calmare treatment as a crossover group. Seven did so and were treated identically to the original two groups except for the elimination of the blind. In the ten-session study, the subjects received an fMRI followed by treatment on day one, treatment only on days two through nine, then treatment followed by an fMRI on day 10. They were scheduled to return for a third fMRI approximately six weeks from the second fMRI. Two subjects were completely relieved of pain before the end of the set of 10 treatments. They were not treated further and did not experience a return of pain before day 10. They also received the second fMRI on day 10. Subjects in the ten-session study were interviewed by phone approximately 12 weeks after the end of treatment (~6 weeks after the third fMRI) about the overall results of the study.

Nerve stimulations instrumentation characteristics

Treatments were administered using a Calmare (Model MC-5A, Competitive Technologies Inc., Seoul, Korea) with two TENS (TENS7000, Current Solutions, LLC, Austin, Texas) units mounted to it on a plexiglass frame (see Figure S1). The amplitude knobs of the TENS units were ganged with those of the Calmare with O-rings and the outputs selected under Bluetooth control (see Figure S2). The TENS unit continuously generates rectangular, unidirectional 300 μs-wide pulses at 43 Hz. The Calmare unit generates distorted sine waves (see Figure S3) with a base frequency varying between 46 and 56 Hz from one random duration period (RDP) to the next, and harmonics that vary in intensity from one RDP to the next (see Figure S4). The harmonics distort the sine wave, and the variation in base frequency and harmonic intensities assure that the distortion changes from one RDP to the next. The RDPs lasted ~2 s on average.

Double-blind management and treatment protocol

Subjects were randomly assigned to therapy groups and the instrument switch was set for each subject by the double-blind supervisor (see Figure S1). The therapist applied the electrodes proximal to the affected area on the seated subject, typically with a pair on each affected limb, and raised the signal amplitude by turning the ganged knob for each lead pair. Subjects were asked to report the level of pain relief as the amplitude was increased to an optimal level. Sometimes the electrodes or the amplitude were further adjusted during the 30-minute treatment period. Subjects rated their pre- and post-treatment pain apart from the therapist either in writing (preliminary study) or using a laptop (ten-session study) using the Washington Neuropathic Pain Scale (WNPS) (11, 12) and the Visual Analog Scale (VAS) (28) each day of treatment, with superficial burning pain reduction pre-specified as the primary outcome. Following therapy, the therapist took notes on electrode placement, area in pain, and other observations.

Post-treatment MRI and follow-up

The subjects returned after one day (one-session study) or approximately six weeks (ten-session study) and again rated their pain using the WNPS and VAS and had MRI scans. In the ten-session study, subjects were also called ~12 weeks after the therapy to verbally rate their pain with the WNPS and other follow-up qualitative questions about the duration of effects, feedback for the study, life events that may have affected the study, and their guess regarding their modality group assignment.

MRI scan parameters

All MRI scans were performed on a Siemens 3T Tim Trio scanner with a 32-channel head coil at the BYU MRI Research Facility. Structural images were acquired using a T1-weighted MPRAGE sequence with the following parameters: TR = 20 ms, TE = 4.92 ms, slices = 192 interleaved, voxel size = 1.0 × 1.0 × 1.0 mm, FOV = 256 mm, flip angle = 25°, total acquisition time = 8:55 min. Resting state BOLD data were acquired using a multi-band EPI sequence with the following parameters: multi-band factor = 8, TR = 867 ms (1125 TRs), TE = 44.2 ms, slices = 72 interleaved, voxel size = 2 × 2 × 2 mm, FOV = 208 mm, flip angle = 52°, total acquisition time = 12:06 min. The first five volumes acquired were discarded to allow for T1 equilibration.

MRI data preprocessing

Preprocessing was performed using the Analysis of Functional Neuroimages (AFNI) suite of programs and Advanced Normalization Tools (ANTs) (29, 30). The following steps were performed: 1) structural and functional image co-registration, 2) de-spiking, 3) motion correction by censoring of image in which there was a significant motion event (>.5 mm translation), 4) noise regression of a) white matter, b) CSF, and c) motion-related noise. Cleaned fMRI time series were segmented according to the Automated Anatomical Labeling Atlas (31) as updated with additional subdivisions of the orbitofrontal cortex, AAL2, (32) after which the 94 region-of-interest (ROI) time signals were averaged within regions and correlated between regions for the creation of a scan-specific correlation matrix.

Analysis of subjective pain reports

Student's t-tests were performed on treatment group averaged VAS and WNPS pain scores. Also, three lines of evidence were combined to assess the pained areas *post hoc* using the definitions in Table 1: 1) patient drawings on the initial interview, 2) therapist drawings at the beginning of treatment sessions, and 3) electrode positioning notes by the therapist.

Table 1. Definitions of pain areas

Pain Regions[a]	Lower Quadrants	Upper Quadrants
Region 1	Toes and either tops or bottoms of feet	Fingers
Region 2	Whole foot up to ankle	Whole hand up to wrist
Region 3	Ankle to knee	Wrist to elbow
Region 4	Knee to groin	Elbow to shoulder dermatomes (C4-T3)
Region 5	Superior to groin (left or right)	Torso (left or right) except shoulder dermatomes

[a]A region was considered "in pain" if a subject reported pain in any portion of that region.

These were used for comparison of proportions and odds-ratio hypothesis testing (details in Supplemental Data: Statistical Methods). To reduce the likelihood of false positive findings due to multiple comparisons, statistical significance for a given test was only considered relevant if it appeared in at least four of the five groups.

Objective fMRI pain analysis methods (correlation and graph theory analysis)

Weighted correlation matrices were produced by correlating the time courses of all pairs of ROIs. For statistical tests performed on these raw correlation matrices, Fisher's R-to-Z transformation was first applied. Then, the treatment effects on ROI-pairing functional connectivity were examined. A subset of 13 paired ROIs commonly implicated in chronic pain, i.e., superior medial prefrontal cortex, orbital medial prefrontal cortex, insula, anterior cingulate gyrus, middle cingulate gyrus, posterior cingulate gyrus, hippocampus, amygdala, precuneus, caudate, putamen, globus pallidum, and thalamus, with $n \times (n-1)/2 = 325$ correlations, was selected for analysis. As pain score changes were largest between scans 1 (pretreatment) and 2 (post treatment in the first study, and post final treatment in the second study), we focused on treatment effects from scan 1 to 2. We performed paired T-tests of treatment effect on the correlation coefficient for each treatment group (Calmare vs TENS vs crossover in the first study; Calmare vs TENS in the second study). Results were considered relevant when the P value was below 0.05 for a given pairing in multiple groups, again out of consideration for possible false positives in any given test in a single group. Additionally, we examined treatment effects on network properties of subject brain correlation-coefficient graphs (i.e., sets of linked nodes, where the nodes are ROIs and the links are correlation coefficients across scans). Weighted correlation matrices were given a threshold at 10% sparsity. Graph measures of connectivity were taken from the Brain Connectivity Toolbox (33) and were implemented in MATLAB (MathWorks Inc, Natick, MA). For each scan, the global efficiency and global modularity were calculated. Then, for each ROI within each scan, the regional metrics of clustering coefficient, degree, and betweenness centrality were determined. Treatment effects on global graph metrics were examined with paired T-tests between scans 1 and 2 in both studies with a significance level set at $\alpha = 0.95$. Graph metrics with significant changes from scan 1 to scan 2 were further examined in a linear mixed-effects regression (the R language LME4 package) as predictors of pain score. fMRI observables were pre-specified as secondary outcome measures.

FINDINGS

Subjective pain score results

The group average VAS and WNPS residual pain scores were substantially reduced relative to the initial scores after the ten-session treatment (see Table 2). The two treatment modalities resulted in similar pain reductions for all pain types, with hot and surface pain being the most reduced types. Average pain scores reported at six weeks after the therapy remained reduced, especially for hot pain and surface pain in both groups, but also for cold pain in the Calmare group and sharp pain and sensitivity in the TENS group. No subject reported increased pain or other unintended effects.

The WNPS hot pain scores in the two studies (see Figure 2), dropped significantly ($P < 0.01$) after the first treatment, with one exception (TENS in the one-session study). There were also significant drops after the first treatment in the WNPS intense pain score in the ten-session study and the VAS scores in both studies (see Figures S5-S7). Pain reductions were not significantly different between TENS and Calmare. The crossover Calmare treatment during the one-session study also produced statistically significant drops in both VAS ($P < 0.01$) (see Figure S6) and WNPS hot pain ($P < 0.01$) (see Figure 2C). In the ten-session study, the WNPS hot pain scores dropped upon the first treatment (see Figure 2, D and E) and then stayed low for the ten-session period for both Calmare and TENS treatments (see Figure 3), with each treatment producing a small effect that was lost by the next day. Both methods of treatment were also successful in reducing pain by the final day (post 10) compared to day 1, ($P < 0.005$). There was no significant difference between Calmare and TENS in total pain reduction (Post 10 vs Pre 1, $P > 0.05$). The return of pain at 6 weeks (pre W6) was modest, the same for the two groups ($P > 0.05$).

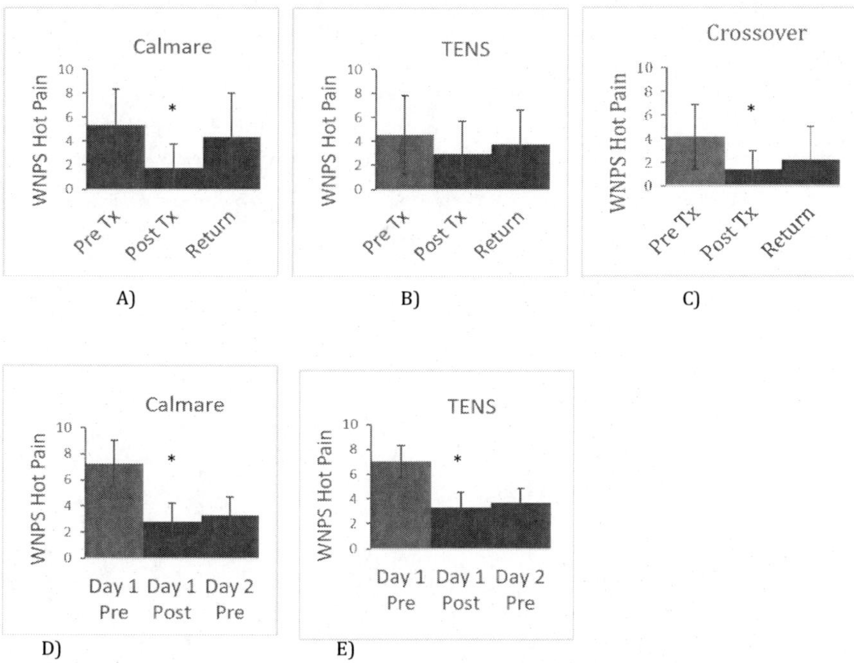

Figure 2. Upper: Average subject hot pain (WNPS) ratings for one-session study before treatment (blue), after treatment (red), and next day (purple) for A) Calmare group (N = 9), B) TENS group (N = 9), and C) Crossover group (N = 7). Error bars are ± 2 S.E.M. *$P < 0.01$ (treatment effect, Post Tx vs Pre Tx, paired, one-tailed T test). Lower: Average subject hot pain (WNPS) ratings for ten-session study before treatment 1 (after fMRI, blue), after treatment 1 (red), and (before treatment) next day (day 2, purple) for D) Calmare group (N = 10), E) TENS group (N = 9). Error bars are ± 2 S.E.M. *$P < 0.01$ (treatment effect, Post Tx vs Pre Tx, paired, one-tailed T test).

Table 2. Average relative[a] pain remaining

	Calmare		*TENS*	
	10 Day Tx	**6 Week Return**	**10 Day Tx**	**6 Week Return**
VAS Pain	38%	93%	15%	69%
WNPS Intense Pain	35%	78%	32%	66%
WNPS Sharp Pain	31%	70%	28%	53%
WNPS Hot Pain	30%	52%	27%	48%
WNPS Dull Pain	51%	73%	39%	70%
WNPS Cold Pain	28%	59%	46%	61%
WNPS Sensitivity	35%	67%	31%	57%
WNPS Itchy Pain	61%	82%	43%	81%
WNPS Unpleasant Pain	43%	84%	33%	71%
WNPS Deep Pain	39%	81%	35%	78%
WNPS Surface Pain	30%	64%	27%	56%

[a]Average pain after ten-session therapy and upon follow-up 6 weeks later relative to the original score. N=8-10 in each case (all subjects completed the initial surveys, but in some cases one survey answer was missed at the end of treatments and two were missed at the 6-week return).

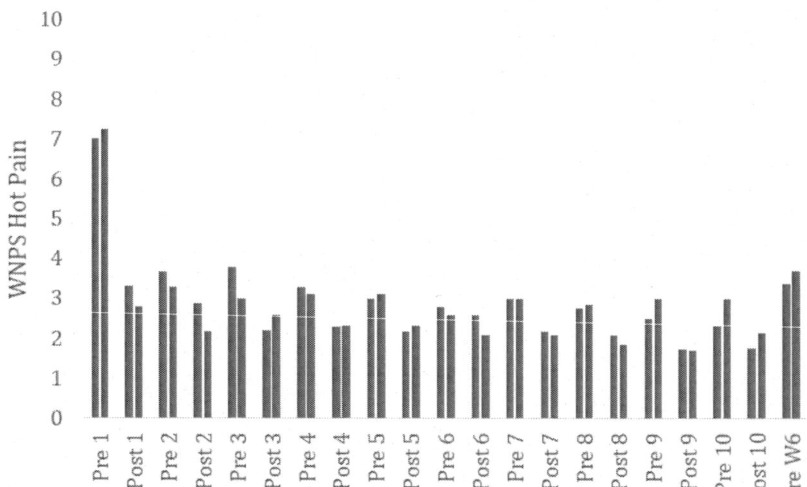

Figure 3. Average subject hot pain (WNPS) ratings for ten-session study before (pre) and after (post) treatment each day and before fMRI at the 6-week post-treatment follow-up for Calmare group (orange, N = 8-10) and TENS group (blue, N = 8-10).

Post hoc subjective pain region results

As shown in Figure 4, the total numbers of pain-affected regions (summed over all the subjects in a group) before the ten-session study were 80 (Calmare) and 51 (TENS). A comparison of proportions test showed the number of pain areas was more effectively reduced by Calmare than by TENS ($Z = 3.19$, $p < 0.005$). Using the same data set, the odds ratio test for treatment success (reduction in number of pained areas to one or zero in a given quadrant) was 22.67 [95% CI 4.71 to 109], with Calmare treatment more effective than TENS ($P < 0.0001$).

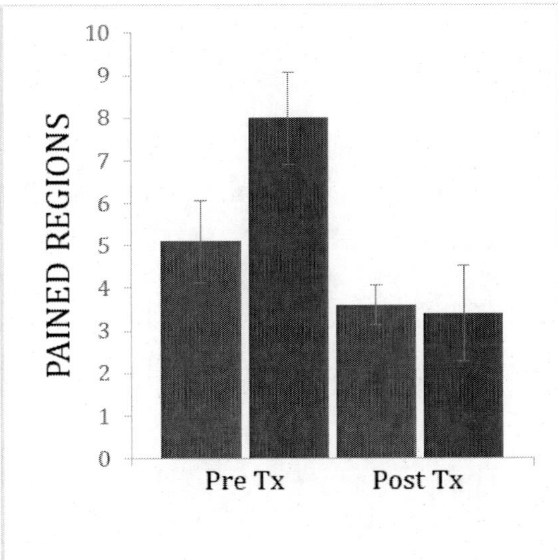

Figure 4. The pre-treatment number of pained regions as compared to the post-treatment total for the Calmare group (red) and the TENS group (blue) in the ten-session study.

fMRI results

T-tests on the Pearson's R Correlation Coefficients, Fisher R-to-Z transformed: The left hippocampus-right amygdala correlation was increased upon treatment ($P < 0.05$) in three of the groups, i.e., Calmare

(0.015 ± 0.13, n = 9 to 0.23 ± 0.22, n = 9) in the one-session study, and both TENS (0.047 ± 0.13, n = 8 to 0.25 ± 0.18, n = 8) and Calmare (0.15 ± 0.16, n = 9 to 0.26 ± 0.14, n = 9) groups from the ten-session study, and increased but possibly underpowered in the TENS one-session study (0.097 ± 0.24, n = 8 to 0.23 ± 0.11, n = 8, $P<0.1$) and decreased slightly in the Crossover study (0.17 ± 0.20, n = 7 to 0.14 ± 0.24, n = 7, $P<0.3$).

Graph theory analysis

No significant differences were observed in any regional graph theory metrics from scan 1 to 2 in either study. We tested for changes in functional brain graph global efficiency from scan 1 to 2. In the one-day study, the crossover group and all groups when combined had increased global efficiency ($p < 0.05$) after treatment. In the two-week study, both treatment groups, when combined, also had significantly increased global efficiency as a result of treatment ($p < 0.05$). In a mixed effects model with global efficiency as a fixed effect predictor of pain score and with subject ID included as a random effect, we found that global efficiency significantly predicted neither VAS nor WNPS intensity pain scores ($p > 0.05$).

Evaluation of the blind

In a perfect blind, the subjects and therapists would predict the assigned treatment group correctly 50% of the time. In the one-session study, 56% of the subjects predicted correctly the day after the treatment along with 72% of the therapists. In the ten-session study, the subjects were 83% correct after the treatments and 69% correct 12 weeks later, while the therapists were 94% correct after the treatments.

Discussion

To our knowledge, this is the first report of a Calmare study of peripheral neuropathy with a double-blind, active TENS control. A similar randomized non-blind study using a TENS control group was carried out during the same period as this study, which showed superiority in Calmare treatment effects compared to TENS treatment effects (34). Here, the Calmare was effective in reducing reported pain scores for a prolonged period in the ten-session paradigm, as was TENS. Calmare was more effective in reducing the number of pained areas. This is plausible because animal and human clinical studies (35) have shown that high frequency (>100 Hz) and low frequency (<10 Hz) TENS have differential effects on descending pain regulation pathways in the spinal cord, suggesting that a mix of non-traditional frequencies, such as found in the Calmare harmonics, could optimize efficacy.

The subject blind was moderately successful, but the therapist blind was quite unsuccessful (see Figure S1 for further discussion). In future studies, single-blind with comparison of traditional TENS and Calmare would be equally successful and easier to administer. The recent study of neuromyelitis optica (10) compared Calmare to a vibrator single-blind and showed significant effects of Calmare and no effect of the vibrator on pain, with good statistical blinding of the subjects. The observation that traditional TENS was equally effective at prolonged block of pain suggests that generic electrical nerve stimulation, but not the vibratory nerve stimulation parameters used there, mediates the pain relief.

In the fMRI studies, global efficiency and left-hippocampus/right-amygdala correlations were increased by treatment. This neural correlate to decreased perception of chronic pain can be interpreted in terms of the "learned pain" model, in which the central circuits subserving acute pain are inappropriately prolonged by learning and memory based in the hippocampus (14, 20, 36). These central circuits include both analytical localization in the somatosensory cortex and affective evaluation in the limbic system (e.g., cingulate gyrus and amygdala). With the expectation that the most likely treatment-effect changes in central function would be in the limbic system (37), we initially searched for reduced activity (blood flow) or connectivity (correlation in the time series of blood flow fluctuations) in these regions. Because the subjective pain reports for the two Calmare, two TENS and one crossover group were similar, we evaluated their fMRI results both independently and jointly. As expected for resting fMRI, the blood flow variations were not statistically significant, and the correlation coefficients showed many possible statistically significant (at $\alpha = 0.05$) interactions between the 13 regions of interest, but none except the left-hippocampus/right-amygdala increase was reproducible between the five groups. Interestingly, the left hippocampal morphology has been recently implicated in biasing memories of pain (38) in ways that can affect personality-dependent placebo responses in chronic pain. Nevertheless, the increased correlation between the left hippocampus and right amygdala upon reduction of pain is difficult to rationalize both because of the contralateral connection, which has no obvious direct neurological basis, and because one might expect such an increase in correlation to subserve aberrant memory of pain, rather than a decrease in pain. One is forced to speculate that the increased correlation in this particular circuit is inhibitory rather than excitatory and of sufficient magnitude as to stand out. In an intra-operative corticocortical evoked potential study of medicinally intractable seizure patients, stimulation of the left posterior hippocampus was found to produce recordable activity in the right posterior cingulate gyrus and stimulation of the right posterior cingulate gyrus produced recordable activity in the right amygdala (39). Perhaps this indirect (two-step) connection between the left hippocampus and right amygdala, obscured by network complexities, is responsible for the increased left hippocampus/right amygdala correlation treatment effect reported here.

Regional network analysis using graph theory, in which each region of interest is treated as a "node" and each pairwise correlation with 93 regions as a possible "edge," yielded no consistent change in any of the standard metrics (see methods). But global efficiency, the connectivity of the global network, was increased after treatment for both studies when the treatment groups were combined. This can be interpreted to suggest that an individual in chronic pain reflexively shuts down many connections in the brain, perhaps as one might expect for a defensive posture where the brain limits its interactions in negative feed-forward preparation for focal risks. Once the risk is perceived as resolved, the brain returns to a more globally free interaction state where it monitors input in a non-selective fashion, prepared for any eventuality of environmental change. After therapy, interactions between regional pairings deemed to be of lower priority for the focal risk are disinhibited and global efficiency returns to a "broad environmental surveillance" state. Correlations between the important limbic regions, the hippocampal "memory" region and the amygdala "fear, reward learning, anxiety" region could reasonably be expected to subserve the learned pain phenotype.

Both the pain and fMRI observations presented here involved multiple measurements. In both cases, the reproducibility of uncorrected statistical significance for given measures between similar groups (TENS and Calmare, one-session and first session of the ten-session) is used as a measure of reliability. It was originally intended that the fMRIs results from the one-session study would allow power estimates for the second study, but ultimately it became expedient to proceed with the ten-session study before that could be accomplished.

In future studies, perhaps connections with the localization regions responsive to the individual subject's specific pained areas (i.e., in "foot region" of the postcentral gyrus) and/or with the error detection regions of the cingulate gyrus (40) could also be identified. Normal (pain-free) treated controls would be valuable to distinguish pain reduction effects from pain-unrelated treatment effects and a single-treatment paradigm would be sufficient.

Conclusion

In conclusion, Calmare and TENS both produced prolonged, substantial pain relief for subjects with idiopathic peripheral neuropathy and fMRI showed increased correlations between blood flow vacillations in left-hippocampus and right-amygdala as well as increased global efficiency after a single treatment session and after a series of ten daily treatments.

Acknowledgments

The authors are grateful to Dale Hardy (Provo, UT, USA) and Eric Bingham (DC, Utah Valley Chiropractic, Pleasant Grove, UT, USA) for inspiring, facilitating, and supporting the studies with time and effort, Bob Hallock (Scientific Support Shop, Brigham Young University, Provo, UT, USA) for designing and building the double blind treatment device, Zac Cetraro, Janai Goodwin, and Seth Parker (Students at Brigham Young University, Provo, UT, USA) for help with subject management, Prof. Brian Mazzeo (Dept of Electrical Engineering, Brigham Young University, Provo, UT, USA) for help with the spectrum analysis of the Calmare output, Paula Johnson (PhD student, Department of Psychology, Brigham Young University, Provo, UT, USA) for help in fMRI scanning, and Assoc. Prof. Brock Kirwan (Dept. of Psychology, Brigham Young University, Provo, UT, USA) for help with data analysis methods. Funding for both studies, including user fees for the Brigham Young University Magnetic Resonance Imaging Research Facility, was provided by the Sorenson Legacy Foundation. Access to the Calmare instrument was by rental from Competitive Technologies for the first study and rental from a private owner for the second study.

SUPPLEMENTAL DATA

Statistical methods

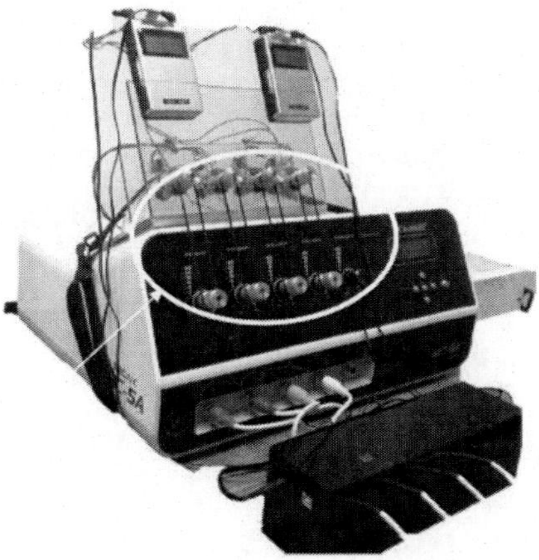

Figure S1. Assembled TENS/Calmare double-blind device. The two TENS units are mounted on plexiglass above the Calmare. The white oval encompasses the O-ring assembly that mechanically couples the amplitude control of the TENS to that of the Calmare. The black box in front contains the Arduino-controlled switch for the output, governing whether the TENS input or the Calmare input is put out. The two TENS devices, each with two independent outputs (top) were modified to have output amplitudes governed by one-turn potentiometers controlled by aluminum knobs. The knobs were mounted on the plexiglass rack. The aluminum knobs were mechanically coupled by O-rings to similar aluminum knobs, which, using set screws, replaced the knobs on the Calmare. The output leads from the TENS and Calmare were both fed into a black plexiglass box containing a Bluetooth receiver (Arduino UNO, Arduino, Somerville, Massachusetts). The receiver was controlled by a computer kept out of the treatment room, or out of sight in the treatment room, to switch all inputs from either the Calmare or the TENS to the four outputs from the black box. Then, each of the knobs was set at the counterclockwise extreme to eliminate any accumulation of slippage of the O-rings between sessions. A trained therapist, blind to the treatment group, then placed up to 4 electrode pairs on the subject's skin proximal to the region of pain. Generally, one pair was applied transversely to each leg or ankle. But in a few cases of foot and hand neuropathy, additional pairs were applied to the wrists. Then, while asking the subject about the level of sensation, the therapist or assistant would turn up the amplitude slowly and gently until the subject reported feeling a mild shock sensation, and then proceeded a bit further until the subject reported cessation of the chronic pain, or until the knob reached its maximum position, which always occurred below the muscle contraction induction level. As the therapist turned up a Calmare knob, the TENS knob controlling the same output lead was rotated an equal amount by the O-ring, producing a signal of similar amplitude, subjectively speaking, whichever of the two modalities was being applied. This double-blind design benefits from simplicity, but suffers from a few unavoidable tells that may become evident to experienced therapists, but still could be easily hidden from subjects. The most apparent tell is that the Calmare signal varies while TENS is steady, which therapists may realize and subjects may inadvertently comment on during electrode placement. A more subtle tell is that the Calmare instrument has, in addition to the broken circuit fault detection, (which this design overcomes, see Figure S2), an undocumented overdrive fault detection which causes it to enter into fault mode occasionally when the amplitude knob is turned nearly all the way up. It seems to be related to circuit resistance, as it seemed to occur more often with some types of electrodes than others and could often be alleviated by replacing the electrodes. We inferred from this behavior that it might be related to a feedback overdrive, such as might be used in a current clamp configuration. The TENS instrument used does not have any fault mode, so a knowledgeable technician might consciously or subconsciously associate Calmare faults with a Calmare group assignment for a given subject.

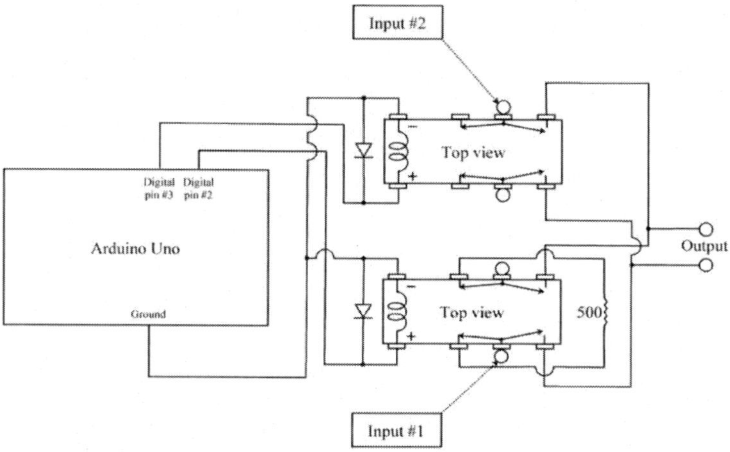

Figure S2. Switching circuitry diagram for assembled TENS/Calmare double blind device. Leads from Calmare and TENS attached to Arduino Uno bluetooth receiver to modulate output through standard electrode pads. The diagram shows the circuitry for one of the four pairs of output leads, all four being controlled simultaneously by the Arduino Uno. Each pair exits the black box in a single cable, which later bifurcates. Circuitry in the switching circuit allowed for each of the four pairs of Calmare leads to be connected through a 500-ohm resistor (simulating skin resistance) when out of the circuit in order to bypass the Calmare broken-circuit detection warning and shut-off. Each input has an inductor connected to a flyback diode, which prevents sudden spikes in voltage across the inductor with sudden interruptions or changes in current. This allows the Arduino Uno to switch which treatment is being administered without disconnecting either of the treatment inputs. The four output leads coming from the black box (initial segments visible in the lower right of Figure S1) were Calmare-brand leads that had been cut, the back ends being inserted as inputs into the black box. The leads were connected to standard electrode pads (Little PALS, Axelgaard Manufacturing Company LTD, Fallbrooke, California) for application to healthy skin regions in the affected limbs of the subjects.

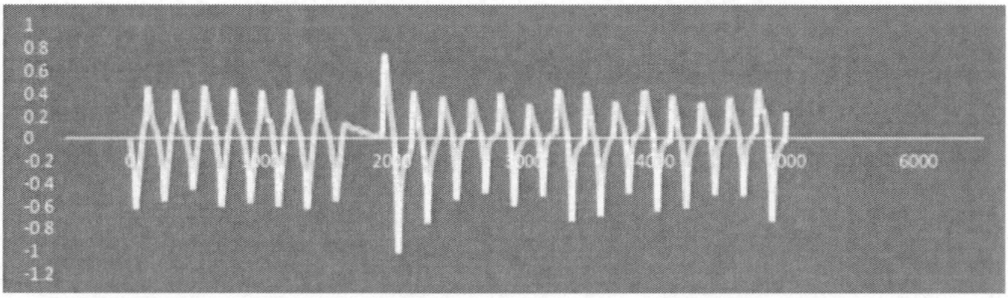

Figure S3. Oscilloscope reading of Calmare output over 0.5 seconds. Analyses of the waveforms generated from the Calmare and TENS units were performed by directly connecting the electrodes to the leads of a digital oscilloscope and spectrum analyzer (Analog Discovery, Discovery Inc., Pullman, Washington). The Calmare output is a randomly distorted sinusoidal curve in contrast to the TENS output, which consists of rectangular pulses with a width of 300 μs initiated and followed by brief double-exponential spikes (not shown) that appear to be designed for charging skin capacitance, such that the ohmic current into the skin is a roughly rectangular pulse.

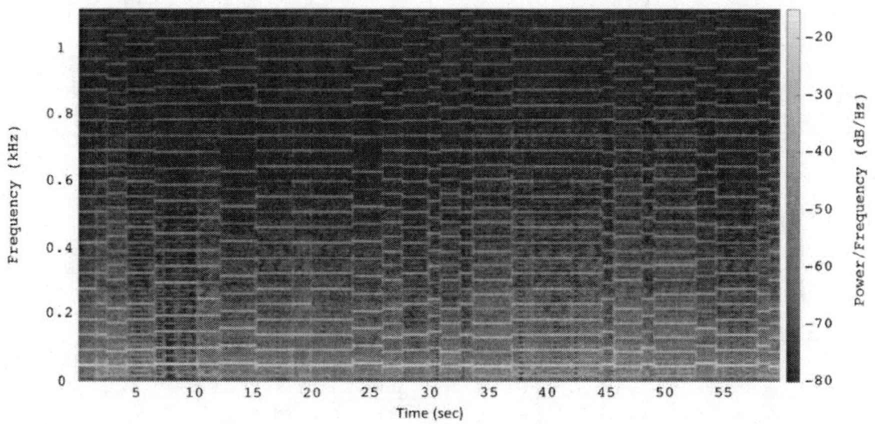

Figure S4. Calmare output spectrogram showing the Fourier transform of Calmare output colorimetrically over a 60 second period. The power amplitude is most intense at the base frequency ~47 Hz) with harmonics of lesser intensity. RDPs are evident as periods of constant base frequency. In each RDP the harmonics of the base frequency have a unique set of intensities.

Table S1. Exclusion criteria

Hospital Anxiety and Depression Scale [1]	Depression score above 15 (severe depression)
MRI criteria	Metal implants or claustrophobia
Maternity status	Pregnancy or breast feeding
Neurological history	History of epilepsy, brain damage, or serious psychiatric disorder (schizophrenia, etc)
Allergies	Skin condition that would preclude placement of electrodes
Therapy history	Neurolytic pain control devices such as implanted spinal cord stimulators used within one month of or during the study

[1] Zigmond AS, Snaith RP. The hospital anxiety and depression scale. Acta Psychiatr Scand. 1983;67(6):361-370.

Table S2. One-treatment study subject characteristics

Sub #	Sex	Age	Dx[1]	Yrs of Pain	Rx[2]	Verbal Pain Description	Drugs
91	F	60	I	10	T	numbness and tingling, no burning pain	-
40	M	51	I	6	C	burning pain	Lyrica BID until 6 weeks ago Ibuprofen PRN (800-1600 mg/day) Flomax & Sudafed PRN.
07	F	35	-	2	C	stabbing pain up Achilles tendon	Lyrica BID for 2 w 1 yr ago Gabapentin for 1 m 1.5 yr ago Metanx BID
02	M	57	D	20	C	pain in bottom of feet and toes	Gabapentin for a few m 4 yrs ago Oxycodone 30 mg TID Tradjenta Metformin Aspirin 325 mg Supplements
09	F	51	I	3	C	neuropathy both feet & hands	Gabapentin 1 qPM for 3 m 1 yr ago

Sub #	Sex	Age	Dx[1]	Yrs of Pain	Rx[2]	Verbal Pain Description	Drugs
36	M	70	I	10	T	no burning pain	Aspirin 81 mg Advil PRN
43	M	59	I	10	T	numbness & tingling, mild burning pain	Gabapentin for 1 m 1.5 yr ago Lyrica BID for 2 w 1 yr ago Metanx BID
64	F	68	D	20+	T	numbness and tingling, no burning pain	Gabapentin 600 mg TID for multiple years until 4-6 w ago Metformin 150 mg TID
16	M	55	I	5-6	T	numbness and tingling, no burning pain	Gabapentin 5-7 pills daily until 3 y ago Sudafed PRN
18	F	71	I	9	T	-	Gabapentin 300 mg PRN, "took one last week," 600 mg TID for 1 w in 2006 Lyrica for several m. in 2006 Levothyroxin 137 mcg qd
51	F	61	I	15	C	burning only in feet	Topamax 50 mg qd Sumatriptan PRN 100 mg for foot pain Naproxen 100 mg BID Celexa 40 mg qd Flexeril 10 mg qd Diphenhydramine (allergy) 25-75 mg qd Valium 10 mg qd Ambien 10 mg qd
53	F	60	I	20	C	numbness, tingling, and burning in both feet	Oxycodone 300 mg q 4h for 3 d 2 m ago. Advil, ibuprofen PRN Synthroid Metformin 250 mg BID Progesterone 100 mg BID
99	F	60	RSD	11	T	burning in upper forearms	Neurontin trial 7 y ago Excedrin PRN migraines Topazepam PRN sleep Atenolol 25 mg qd

Table S2. (Continued)

Sub #	Sex	Age	Dx[1]	Yrs of Pain	Rx[2]	Verbal Pain Description	Drugs
37	M	67	S	20+	C	lumbar pain L5-S1 sciatica bilateral into feet pain mostly on lateral sides of legs	
38	M	59	I	3	C	pain in toes and balls of feet	
50	F	66	C	4	T	numbness & tingling in both feet	
73	M	57	D	10+	T	no burning pain reported	Gabapentin TID Oct 2014-Feb 2015 Lyrica 3-4 y ago Insulin (short and long lasting) Metformin Drugs for acid reflux, high cholesterol, and high blood pressure
20	M	60	D	3	C	numbness & tingling	Milxicam PRN pain Tylenol 650 mg PRN pain Peroxetine Metformin Glimeperide Losartan Claritin D 24-Hr Multivitamin

[1]Peripheral Neuropathy Diagnosis – self-reported: I, idiopathic; D, diabetic; C, Chemotherapy-induced; S, spinal injury; RSD, reflex sympathetic dystrophy; [2]Treatment group: T, TENS; C, Calmare. Summary: Average female age was 59.1 (35-71) years and average male age was 59.4 (51-70). 55.6% of the subjects reported an idiopathic type of peripheral neuropathy, 22.2% reported diabetic, and 22.2% of the subjects were distributed amongst chemotherapy-induced, spinal injury, RSD, and undefined diagnoses. Pain duration ranged from 2 to over 20 years. Although the intent was to gather subjects with burning pain in the extremities and with limited anti-seizure pain med exposure, many of the subjects reported no pain, just numbness and tingling upon arrival for the study.

Table S3. Ten-treatment study subject characteristics

Sub#	Sex	Age	Dx1	Yrs of Pain	Rx2	Verbal Pain Description	Drugs
44	M	65	I	10	C	Dull ache in muscles, tender pressure points, stabbing pain, burning in feet	
41	M	37	D	17	T	Feet keep getting tired, discomfort walking on objects.	
21	F	62	I	15	C	Burning	
59	M	38	C	2	C	Feet started to feel pain and have increased ever since	
54	M	58	D	13	T	Shooting and deep, in feet and then in thigh. A little bit in hands.	Gabapentin (not in 2 weeks)
23	M	71	I	12	C	Pins and needles on surface of toes and bottom of feet	
88	M	64	I	20	T	Keeps him awake	Tramadol (not in 2 weeks)
82	M	67	I	12	C	Pins and needles, numbness and tingling on feet	
65	F	52	H	13	C	Begins in hands and spreads	Lyrica
12	M	60	H	10	T	Begins in feet	
37	F	68	I	4	T	Pain in both feet and legs	
62	F	36	D	5	T	Stinging, hot and cold simultaneously	Gabapentin (not in 2 weeks)
48	F	68	D	5	C	Stinging, burning pain in toes and feet.	
19	F	55	D	3	T	Numb, sharp pain on toes. Cold, like bugs crawling	Gabapentin (not in 2 weeks)
42	M	61	I	3	T	Numb, sharp pain in toes	
33	M		I	15	C	Burning Pain on feet, shins, and hand	
74	F	55	I	2	T	Feet and ankles	Lyrica
00	F	39	C*	8	C	Left side all the way through arm and back	Tramadol

Table S3. (Continued)

Sub#	Sex	Age	Dx1	Yrs of Pain	Rx2	Verbal Pain Description	Drugs
15	F	68	I	-	T	Burning pain on tops and bottoms of feet	Gabapentin
01	F	44	S	24	C	Sharp, burning pain in left foot	

[1]Peripheral Neuropathy Diagnosis – self-reported: I, idiopathic; D, diabetic; C, Chemotherapy-induced; C*, Chronic Regional Pain Syndrome; S, spinal injury; H, Hereditary Sensory Neuropathy; RSD, reflex sympathetic dystrophy; [2]Treatment group: T, TENS; C, Calmare. Summary: The average female age was 54.7 (36-68) years and male age 58.5 (37-67) years. 50% of the subjects reported an idiopathic diagnosis, 25% reported diabetic, and the other 25% were distributed amongst chemotherapy-induced, spinal injury, CRPS, and hereditary diagnoses. Most subjects had dealt with chronic pain for over 5 years, and the majority over 10 years. In this ten-treatment study, more care was taken than in the preliminary study in pre-screening the subjects for pain; also for medication use, although detail was only gathered on anti-seizure or opioid analgesic medications. 60% reported never having used anti-seizure or opioid analgesic medication. Twenty percent had terminated use of gabapentin or tramadol two weeks prior to the study and the remaining 20% terminated Lyrica, gabapentin or tramadol use 0-2 days prior to the study.

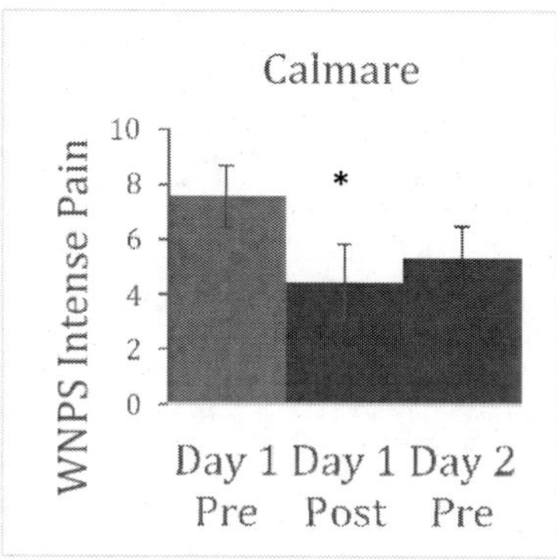

A)

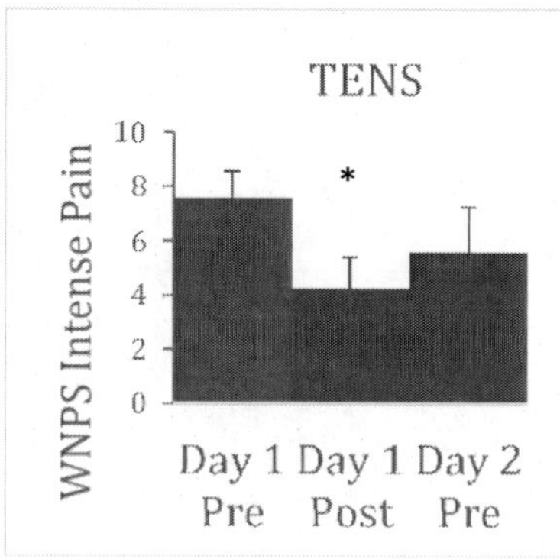

B)

Figure S5. Average intense pain (WNPS) ratings for ten-treatment study before first treatment (after fMRI), after first treatment, and (before second treatment) next day for A)

Calmare group *P < 0.01 (treatment effect, Post Tx (N = 10) vs Pre Tx (N = 8), unpaired, one-tailed T test), B) TENS group (N = 9) *P < 0.01 (treatment effect, Post Tx vs Pre Tx, paired, one-tailed T test). Error bars are ± 2 S.E.M.

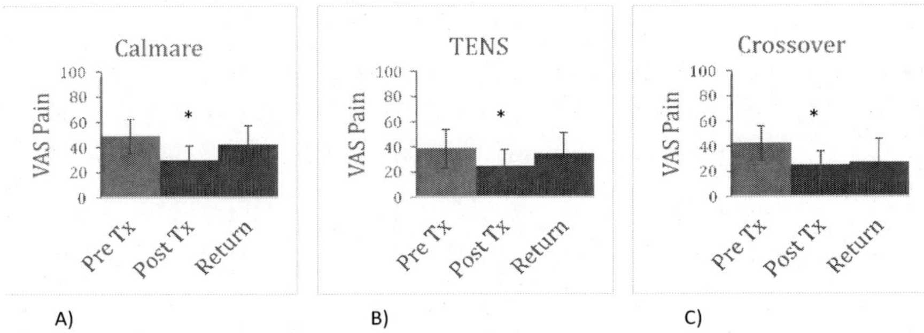

Figure S6. Average subject Visual Analog Scale (VAS) pain ratings in mm for single-treatment study before treatment, after treatment, and next day for A) Calmare group (N = 9) *P < 0.05 (treatment effect, Post Tx vs Pre Tx, paired, one-tailed T test), B) TENS group (N = 9) *P < 0.01 (treatment effect, Post Tx vs Pre Tx, paired, one-tailed T test), and C) Crossover group (N = 8), *P < 0.01 (treatment effect, Post Tx vs Pre Tx, paired, one-tailed T test). Error bars are ± 2 S.E.M.

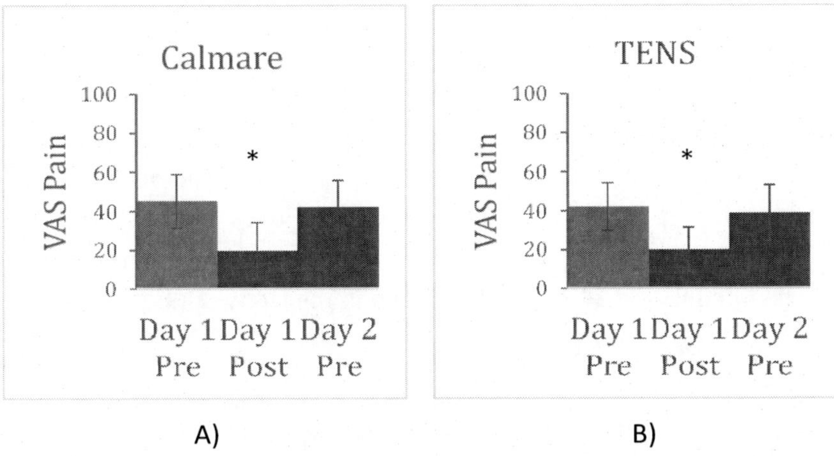

Figure S7. Average subject VAS pain ratings in mm for ten-treatment study before first treatment (after fMRI), after first treatment, and (before second treatment) next day for A) Calmare group *P < 0.05 (treatment effect, Post Tx (N = 10) vs Pre Tx (N = 9), unpaired, one-tailed T test), B) TENS group *P < 0.05 (treatment effect, Post Tx (N = 9) vs Pre Tx (N = 10), paired, one-tailed T test). Error bars are ± 2 S.E.M.

Statistical methods

Comparison of proportions

For each group, the proportion of interest was defined as the number of regions relieved of pain after treatment relative to the total number of pained regions before treatment. The difference in the proportions of relieved pain regions for the Calmare group ($\bar{P}_1$) and TENS group ($\bar{P}_2$) relative to the composite standard error (which is based on the composite proportion of pained regions ($\bar{P}$) and the initial pain region counts for the Calmare group (n_1) and the TENS group (n_2)) was assumed to be Z distributed (Eq. 1) for the hypothesis test.

$$Z = \frac{(\bar{p}_1 - \bar{p}_2)}{\sqrt{\bar{p}(1-\bar{p})\left(\frac{1}{n_1}+\frac{1}{n_2}\right)}} \qquad (1)$$

Odds ratio

The treatment of each affected subject-quadrant (as defined in Table 1) was determined to be "success" if only one region in the quadrant was still affected post-treatment or the quadrant was completely pain free. Otherwise, the treatment was classified as "failure." The odds ratio (OR) is defined in Eq. 2 and its standard error in Eq. 3 where a, b, c, and d represent Calmare "success" count, Calmare "failure" count, TENS "success" count, and TENS "failure" count, respectively. Equation 4 gives the 95% confidence interval for OR.

$$OR = \frac{Calmare\ Success \times Tens\ Failure}{Calmare\ Failure \times Tens\ Success} \qquad (2)$$

$$SE(OR) = \sqrt{\frac{1}{a}+\frac{1}{b}+\frac{1}{c}+\frac{1}{d}} \qquad (3)$$

$$CI \equiv e^{(\log(OR) \pm [1.96 \times SE(\log(OR))])} \qquad (4)$$

REFERENCES

[1] Jin DM, Xu Y, Geng DF, Yan TB. Effect of transcutaneous electrical nerve stimulation on symptomatic diabetic peripheral neuropathy: a meta-analysis of randomized controlled trials. Diabetes Res Clin Pract 2010;89(1):10-5.

[2] Kilinc M, Livanelioglu A, Yildirim SA, Tan E. Effects of transcutaneous electrical nerve stimulation in patients with peripheral and central neuropathic pain. J Rehabil Med 2014;46(5):454-60.

[3] Norrbrink C. Transcutaneous electrical nerve stimulation for treatment of spinal cord injury neuropathic pain. J Rehabil Res Dev 2009;46(1):85-93.

[4] Celik EC, Erhan B, Gunduz B, Lakse E. The effect of low-frequency TENS in the treatment of neuropathic pain in patients with spinal cord injury. Spinal Cord 2013;51(4):334-7.

[5] Majithia N, Smith TJ, Coyne PJ, Abdi S, Pachman DR, Lachance D, et al. Scrambler therapy for the management of chronic pain. Support Care Cancer 2016;24(6):2807-14.

[6] Smith T, Cheville AL, Loprinzi CL, Longo-Schoberlein D. Scrambler therapy for the treatment of chronic post-mastectomy pain (cPMP). Cureus 2017;9(6):e1378.

[7] Smith TJ, Razzak AR, Blackford AL, Ensminger J, Saiki C, Longo-Schoberlein, D, et al. A pilot randomized sham-controlled trial of MC5-A scrambler therapy in the treatment of chronic chemotherapy-induced peripheral neuropathy (CIPN). J Palliat Care 2020;35(1):53-8.

[8] Pachman DR, Weisbrod BL, Seisler DK, Barton DL, Fee-Schroeder KC, Smith TJ, et al. Pilot evaluation of Scrambler therapy for the treatment of chemotherapy-induced peripheral neuropathy. Support Care Cancer 2015;23(4):943-51.

[9] Coyne PJ, Wan W, Dodson P, Swainey C, Smith TJ. A trial of Scrambler therapy in the treatment of cancer pain syndromes and chronic chemotherapy-induced peripheral neuropathy. J Pain Palliat Care Pharmacother 2013;27(4):359-64.

[10] Mealy MA, Kozachik SL, Cook, LJ, Totonis L, Salazar RA, Allen JK, et al. Scrambler therapy improves pain in neuromyelitis optica: A randomized controlled trial. Neurology 2020;94:e1900-7. doi:10.1212/WNL0000000000009370.

[11] Galer BS, Jensen MP. Development and preliminary validation of a pain measure specific to neuropathic pain: the Neuropathic Pain Scale. Neurology 1997;48:332-8.

[12] Jensen MP, Friedman M, Bonzo D, Richards P. The validity of the neuropathic pain scale for assessing diabetic neuropathic pain in a clinical trial. Clin J Pain 2006;22(1):97-103.

[13] Wager TD, Atlas LY, Lindquist MA, Roy M, Woo C-W, Kross E. An fMRI-Based Neurologic Signature of Physical Pain. New England Journal of Medicine. 2013;368(15):1388-97.

[14] Apkarian AV, Baliki MN, Geha PY. Towards a theory of chronic pain. Prog Neurobiol 2009;87(2):81-97.

[15] Baliki MN, Schnitzer TJ, Bauer WR, Apkarian AV. Brain morphological signatures for chronic pain. PLoS One 2011;6(10):e26010.

[16] Malinen S, Vartiainen N, Hlushchuk Y, et al. Aberrant temporal and spatial brain activity during rest in patients with chronic pain. Proc Natl Acad Sci USA 2010;107(14):6493-7.

[17] Bolwerk A, Seifert F, Maihofner C. Altered resting-state functional connectivity in complex regional pain syndrome. J Pain 2013;14(10):1107-15.

[18] Simons LE, Pielech M, Erpelding N, Linnman C, Moulton E, Sava W, et al. The responsive amygdala: treatment-induced alterations in functional connectivity in pediatric complex regional pain syndrome. Pain 2014;155(9):1727-42.

[19] Baliki MN, Mansour AR, Baria AT, Apkarian AV. Functional reorganization of the default mode network across chronic pain conditions. PLoS One 2014;9(9):e106133.

[20] Vachon-Presseau E, Centeno MV, Ren W, Berger SE, Tétreault P, Ghantous M, et al. The emotional brain as a predictor and amplifier of chronic pain. J Dent Res 2016;95(6):605-12.

[21] Borsook D, Becerra LR. Breaking down the barriers: fMRI applications in pain, analgesia and analgesics. Mol Pain 2006;2:30.

[22] Cauda F, Sacco K, Duca S, Cocito D, D'Agata F, Geminiani GC, et al. Altered resting state in diabetic neuropathic pain. PLoS One 2009;4(2):e4542.

[23] Wager TD, Atlas LY, Leotti LA, Rilling JK. Predicting individual differences in placebo analgesia: contributions of brain activity during anticipation and pain experience. J Neurosci 2011;31(2):439-52.

[24] Vachon-Presseau E, Berger SE, Abdullah TB, Huang L, Cecchi GA, Griffith JW, et al. Brain and psychological determinants of placebo pill response in chronic pain patients. Nat Commun 2018;9(1):3397.

[25] Atlas LY, Wielgosz J, Whittington RA, Wager TD. Specifying the non-specific factors underlying opioid analgesia: expectancy, attention, and affect. Psychopharmacology (Berl) 2014;231(5):813-23.

[26] Sevel LS, O'Shea AM, Letzen JE, Craggs JG, Price DD, Robinson ME. Effective connectivity predicts future placebo analgesic response: A dynamic causal modeling study of pain processing in healthy controls. Neuroimage 2015;110:87-94.

[27] Tetreault P, Baliki MN, Baria AT, Bauer WR, Schnitzer TJ, Apkarian AV. Inferring distinct mechanisms in the absence of subjective differences: Placebo and centrally acting analgesic underlie unique brain adaptations. Hum Brain Mapp 2018;39(5):2210-23.

[28] Hawker GA, Mian S, Kendzerska T, French M. Measures of adult pain: Visual Analog Scale for Pain (VAS Pain), Numeric Rating Scale for Pain (NRS Pain), McGill Pain Questionnaire (MPQ), Short-Form McGill Pain Questionnaire (SF-MPQ), Chronic Pain Grade Scale (CPGS), Short Form-36 Bodily Pain Scale (SF-36

BPS), and Measure of Intermittent and Constant Osteoarthritis Pain (ICOAP). Arthritis Care Res (Hoboken) 2011;63(Suppl 11):S240-52.

[29] Cox RW. AFNI: Software for analysis and visualization of functional magnetic resonance neuroimages. Comput Biomed Res 1996;29(3):162-73.

[30] Klein A, Andersson J, Ardekani BA, Ashburner J, Avants B, Chiang MC, et al. Evaluation of 14 nonlinear deformation algorithms applied to human brain MRI registration. Neuroimage 2009;46(3):786-802.

[31] Tzourio-Mazoyer N, Landeau B, Papathanassiou D, Crivello F, Etard O, Delcroix N, et al. Automated anatomical labeling of activations in SPM using a macroscopic anatomical parcellation of the MNI MRI single-subject brain. Neuroimage 2002;15(1):273-89.

[32] Rolls ET, Joliot M, Tzourio-Mazoyer N. Implementation of a new parcellation of the orbitofrontal cortex in the automated anatomical labeling atlas. Neuroimage 2015;122:1-5.

[33] Rubinov M, Sporns O. Complex network measures of brain connectivity: uses and interpretations. Neuroimage 2010;52(3):1059-69.

[34] Loprinzi C, Le-Rademacher JG, Majithia N, McMurray RP, O'Neill CR, Bendel MA, et al. Scrambler therapy for chemotherapy neuropathy: A randomized phase II pilot trial. Support Care Cancer 2020;28(3):1183-97.

[35] Vance CG, Dailey DL, Rakel BA, Sluka KA. Using TENS for pain control: the state of the evidence. Pain Manag 2014;4(3):197-209.

[36] Borsook D, Sava S, Becerra L. The pain imaging revolution: advancing pain into the 21st century. Neuroscientist 2010;16(2):171-85.

[37] Borsook D, Becerra L, Hargreaves R. Biomarkers for chronic pain and analgesia. Part 2: how, where, and what to look for using functional imaging. Discov Med 2011;11(58):209-19.

[38] Berger SE, Vachon-Presseau E, Abdullah TB, Baria AT, Schnitzer TJ, Apkarian AV. Hippocampal morphology mediates biased memories of chronic pain. Neuroimage 2018;166:86-98.

[39] Enatsu R, Gonzalez-Martinez J, Bulacio J, Kubota Y, Mosher J, Burgess RC, et al. Connections of the limbic network: a corticocortical evoked potentials study. Cortex 2015;62:20-33.

[40] Averbeck BB. Unbelievable: Neural correlate of the feedback negativity in the anterior cingulate. Neuron 2017;95(2):237-9.

In: Pain Management
Editors: J Merrick and M Morad
ISBN: 978-1-68507-493-7

Chapter 14

PATIENTS UNDERGOING TREATMENT FOR ORAL CAVITY CANCER AND USE OF OPIOID

Huaising C Ko[1], MD, Mandira N Mehra[2], MD, Adam R Burr[1], MD, Aaron M Wieland[3], MD, Randall J Kimple[1], MD, PhD, Gregory K Hartig[3], MD, Paul M Harari[1], MD and Matthew E Witek[1,4,*], MD, MS

[1]Department of Human Oncology, University of Wisconsin, School of Medicine and Public Health, Madison, Wisconsin, United States of America
[2]Department of Pain Management, SSM Health St. Mary's Hospital, Madison, Wisconsin, United States of America
[3]Department of Surgery, Division of Otolaryngology and Head and Neck Surgery, University of Wisconsin School of Medicine and Public Health, Madison, Wisconsin, United States of America
[4]Department of Radiation Oncology, University of Maryland, School of Medicine, Baltimore, Maryland, United States of America

[*] ***Correspondence:*** Matthew E Witek, MD, MS, 22 South Greene Street, Baltimore, MD 21201, United States. ORCID: 0000-0003-0570-3293. Email: matthew.witek@umm.edu.

Abstract

In the context of the opioid epidemic, there is value in examining the use of opioids in specific cancer patient cohorts. We analyzed opioid use in patients undergoing adjuvant therapy for oral cavity cancer to define the incidence of new persistent use beyond three months. Study Design: Retrospective. Setting: Comprehensive academic cancer center. Subjects and Methods: We performed a retrospective IRB-approved analysis of opioid use in patients who received adjuvant radiotherapy with or with concurrent systemic therapy for surgically resected oral cavity cancer between 2003 and 2016. Factors associated with opioid use were evaluated by Chi-square test and one-way ANOVA. The Kaplan-Meier method was used to estimate overall survival. Results: Of 77 identified patients, 10 (13%) patients received opioid prescriptions at 3 months or greater following completion of radiotherapy. Patients who were opioid naive prior to surgery required significantly fewer opioid prescriptions than intermittent or chronic opioid users. No specific factors were associated with new persistent opioid use. Conclusions: Patients undergoing surgery and adjuvant radiotherapy for oral cavity cancer who required opioids for cancer treatment related pain are at minimal risk for new dependency. Judicious pain management should be applied for patients with a history of prior opioid use. Larger patient cohorts will be needed to identify patient, disease, and treatment characteristics associated with new persistent use given its limited incidence.

Introduction

The prevalence of pain at time of diagnosis for patients with cancers of the head and neck has been estimated at 40-84% (1-5) with the highest pain intensity reported by those with advanced disease with primary tumors of the oral cavity and oropharynx (5, 6). Heterogeneity of tumor burden, proximity and access to cranial nerves, variation in the extent of surgical resection, and differences in pain evaluation have revealed a range of acute post-operative pain assessments ranging from 30-76% (7, 8). In the chronic setting, 25% of patients will report pain for up to at least 2 years after surgery (1).

Opioids are the cornerstone of management of severe pain in patients with cancer (9). A comprehensive study of opioid use for pain control in patients undergoing surgery for non-head and neck malignancies demonstrated new persistent opioid use in 7-11% and 15-21% in patients not receiving or receiving adjuvant chemotherapy, respectively (10). Similarly, evaluation of chronic opioid use in patients with various head and neck cancers undergoing curative intent therapy was 13% (11). The diversity of patient and disease characteristics as well as differences in treatment in these studies limits their applicability to specific disease sites, which maintain distinct patient characteristics, tumor-related pain syndromes, and treatment-induced toxicities.

Given the severity of pain associated with head and neck cancers, especially advanced tumors of the oral cavity, this patient population has a high likelihood of being prescribed opioids for long periods throughout their management. This raises the potential risk of creating opioid dependence. Indeed, a recent retrospective study reported chronic opioid use in 41% of patients undergoing curative surgery for oral cavity squamous cell carcinoma (OCSCC) (12). Furthermore, the addition of adjuvant radiotherapy with or without chemotherapy following surgery for OCSCC may intensify and prolong the pain related to cancer treatment and increases the number of potential prescribers. Thus, this population of patients is a selected subset of individuals at higher risk of becoming new persistent opioid users.

Time from surgery to completion of RT is associated with overall survival in patients with OCSCC (13-16). Therefore, the use of narcotics to optimize pain control in order to prevent treatment delays may play a role in patient outcomes. In light of the conflicting priorities of minimizing the potential for new persistent opioid use and controlling pain to enable timely completion of cancer therapy, we evaluated the use of opioids in patients undergoing adjuvant therapy following curative-intent surgery for OCSCC.

OUR STUDY

We performed an IRB-approved retrospective analysis of opioid prescribing patterns and clinical outcomes of patients identified in our institutional head and neck cancer database who received adjuvant radiotherapy with or without concurrent systemic therapy for resected OCSCC between 2003 and 2016. Patient and disease characteristics, including smoking and alcohol use, treatments rendered, and clinical outcomes were obtained from the database. Patients' electronic medical records were reviewed to collect information regarding type of opioid prescribed, the number and dates of prescriptions, and the number of providers. Patients whose narcotic use was documented in the physician note but not recorded in their electronic medical record with dates of initiation and/or completion were excluded from analysis.

Opioid use

Patients were categorized as naïve, intermittent, or chronic users of opioids, using previously published criteria (10). Opioid naïve patients were defined as those who had no opioid prescriptions between 12 months and 31 days prior to surgery. Patients who were chronic users were those that filled at least 120 days' worth of supply between 12 months and 31 days prior to surgery or documented at least 3 prescriptions in the 90 days prior to surgery. Intermittent users were those whose narcotic prescription pattern fell between naïve and chronic users. Narcotic use was presumed to be associated with cancer treatment and management was designated as prescriptions written within 30 days pre-operatively, as well as those during and 30 days immediately after radiotherapy. Persistent opioid use was defined as consecutive prescription dates no longer than 2 months apart. New persistent opioid use was defined as consecutive prescriptions written 90 days after completion of radiotherapy in patients who were previously opioid naïve.

Statistical analysis

Chi-square test and one-way ANOVA were used to test independence of association between patient factors and opioid use. The Kaplan-Meier method was used to estimate overall survival.

Table 1. Baseline patient and treatment characteristics

Patient Characteristics	Number, (%)
Age (median)	61 years
Sex	
Male	45 (58)
Female	32 (42)
Oral cavity subsite	
Alveolar ridge	12 (15.6)
Buccal mucosa	7 (9.1)
Floor of mouth	15 (19.5)
Hard palate	1 (1.3)
Lip	1 (1.3)
Oral tongue	32 (41.6)
Retromolar trigone	9 (11.7)
T-stage (AJCC 7th edition)	
T1	11 (14.3)
T2	19 (24.7)
T3	4 (5.2)
T4	43 (55.8)
N-stage (AJCC 7th edition)	
N0	29 (37.7)
N1	7 (9.1)
$N2^a$	0 (0)
$N2^b$	32 (41.6)
$N2^c$	9 (11.7)
N3	0 (0)
Type of narcotic user	
[a]Naïve	69 (89.6)
[b]Intermittent	6 (7.8)
[c]Chronic	2 (2.6)
Tobacco (smoking) history	
Non-smoker	21 (27.3)
Current smoker or quit < 1 month prior	33 (42.9)
Quit > 1 month prior	1 (1.3)
Quit > 1 year prior	4 (5.2)
Quit > 5 years prior	4 (5.2)

Table 1. (Continued)

Patient Characteristics	Number, (%)
Quit > 15 years prior	13 (16.9)
No data on smoking history	1 (1.3)
Pack-years, mean (s.d.)	31.1 (32.8)
Alcohol history	
None	2 (2.6)
[d]Social	24 (30.8)
[e]Consistent	16 (20.5)
[f]High volume	19 (24.4)
Previously high but now none	6 (7.7)
No data on alcohol use	11 (14.1)
Radiation dose (median)	63 Gy
Type of Adjuvant Therapy	
Adjuvant radiotherapy	51 (66.2)
Adjuvant chemoradiotherapy	26 (33.8)

Source: [a]no opioid prescription between 12 and 1 months prior to surgery, [b]between naïve and chronic, [c]opioid prescription filled at least 12 and 1 month prior to surgery or filled at least 3 prescriptions in the 3 months prior to surgery, [d]0-6 drinks per week, [e]7-20 drinks per week, [f]21 or more drinks per week.

FINDINGS

We identified 77 patients with OCSCC managed with curative intent surgery (see Table 1). Fifty-one (66.2%) patients received adjuvant RT and 27 patients (34.6%) were managed with adjuvant chemoradiotherapy. The median follow-up was 36.9 months (range 5.5–117.5 months). Oral tongue was the most common oral cavity subsite (41%). The majority of patients had pT4 disease (57%) and were node positive (62%). Tobacco smoking and alcohol use was reported by 70% and 83% of patients, respectively. Nearly 90% of patients were opioid naïve.

Among patients that were naïve, intermittent, or chronic opioid users prior to surgery, there was a positive correlative relationship with the number of prescriptions provided during treatment, as well as the duration of opioid use. There was also a difference in the time from surgery to initiation of adjuvant therapy between these three groups of patients. We did not detect a relationship between the groups with respect to the number of prescription providers, nor in the duration of adjuvant therapy (see Table 2).

Table 2. Impact of prior opioid use on future opioid prescriptions and radiotherapy timing

	All patients median (range)	Naïve median (range)	Intermittent median (range)	Chronic median (range)	p-value
Number of scripts	4 (1-50)	3 (1-31)	7 (1-50)	15 (13-16)	0.03
Duration of opioid use (days)	54 (1-532)	37 (1-532)	110 (1-474)	289 (265-313)	0.03
Number of providers	2 (1-15)	2 (1-15)	5 (1-120	5 (5-5)	0.07
Time from surgery to start of RT	49 (21-107)	49 (21-107)	41 (35-58)	81 (78-84)	0.03
Duration of RT (days)	42 (32-65)	42 (32-65)	42.5 (41-63)	41.5 (39-44)	0.41

Source: RT, radiotherapy.

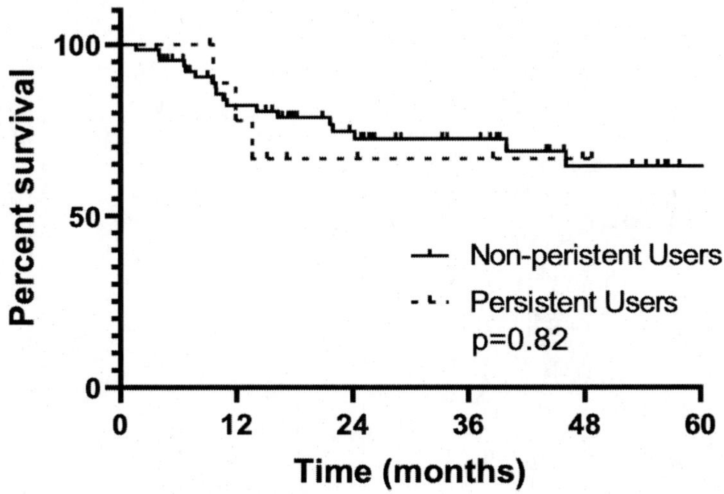

Figure 1. Overall survival for non-persistent users and new persistent opioids users.

Table 3. Association of non-opioid related factors and new persistent opioid use

	Not persistent number, (%)	**New Persistent Number, (n)**	**p-value**
Oral cavity subsite			0.73
Alveolar ridge	12 (17.9)	0 (0)	
Buccal mucosa	6 (8.9)	1 (10)	
Floor of mouth	12 (17.9)	3 (30)	
Hard palate	1 (1.5)	0 (0)	
Lip	1 (1.5)	0 (0)	
Oral tongue	27 (40.3)	5 (50)	
Retromolar trigone	8 (11.9)	1 (10)	
T-stage (AJCC 7th edition)			0.73
T1	9 (13.4)	2 (20)	
T2	17 (25.4)	2 (20)	
T3	3 (4.5)	1 (10)	
T4	38 (56.7)	5 (50)	
N-stage (AJCC 7th edition)			0.73
N0	25 (37.3)	4 (40)	
N1	6 (8.9)	1 (10)	
N2[a]	0(0)	0 (0)	
N2[b]	28 (41.8)	4 (40)	
N2[c]	8 (11.9)	1 (10)	
N3	0 (0)	0 (0)	
Tobacco (smoking) history			0.184
Non-smoker	21 (31.8)	0 (0)	
Current smoker or quit < 1 month prior	26 (39.4)	7 (70)	
Quit > 1 month prior	1 (1.5)	0 (0)	
Quit > 1 year prior	4 (6.1)	0 (0)	
Quit > 5 years prior	4 (6.1)	0 (0)	
Quit > 15 years prior	10 (15.2)	3 (30)	
Alcohol history			0.41
None	2 (3.4)	1 (10)	
Social	22 (37.3)	2 (20)	
Consistent	15 (25.4)	1 (10)	
High volume	16 (27.1)	3 (30)	
Previously high but now none	4 (6.8)	2 (20)	
Adjuvant treatment			0.73
Radiotherapy	44 (65.7)	6 (60)	
Chemoradiotherapy	23 (34.3)	4 (40)	
Type of neck dissection			0.68
None	3 (4.4)	0 (0)	
Unilateral	54 (79.4)	(90)	
Bilateral	11 (16.2)	1 (10)	

Of the entire 77 patient cohort, 13% (n=10) of patients were new persistent users, all of which were opioid naïve, none being prior intermittent users. There were no significant associations between new persistent opioid use and primary tumor site, smoking history, alcohol consumption, T-stage, N-stage, type of adjuvant therapy (radiotherapy versus chemoradiotherapy) or type of neck dissection (bilateral versus unilateral) (see Table 3). Estimated 3-year overall survival for non-persistent users was 64.5% (95% CI: 47.8%-75.5%) and new persistent opioids users was 66.7% (95% CI: 28.2%-87.8%) (p = 0.82) (see Figure 1).

CONCLUSION

The time from initiation of adjuvant RT following surgery (14) and the duration of adjuvant RT (13) impacts the clinical outcomes of patients with OCSCC. Moreover, time from surgery to completion of adjuvant therapy of greater than 14 weeks has been associated with worse overall survival (17). A significant challenge to achieving these goals is adequate pain management. Beyond topical and over-the-counter oral analgesics, opioids form the foundation for severe pain management (9). Retrospective reviews have reported that the most severe pain for patients with head and neck cancers is associated with advanced disease especially arising from primary tumors of the oral cavity (5, 6). Given the potential addicting properties of opioids combined with pain management needs, patients with OCSCC undergoing surgery and adjuvant therapy are at risk for developing long term opioid dependency.

In the present study, we demonstrate that the percentage of patients continuing opioids at three months or greater following completion of radiotherapy was 13%. This is similar to data found in cancer patients undergoing treatment for head and neck cancers from various primary tumor sites (11) as well as therapy for malignancies arising in other anatomic sites (10). Patients that were opioid naive prior to treatment were prescribed significantly less opioids than those with a prior history of opioid prescriptions. There was a difference in time from surgery to initiation of adjuvant therapy amongst patients that were either naïve, intermittent, and chronic opioid users. This was driven by pre-surgery chronic pain patients who represented < 3% of the entire cohort making it difficult to draw conclusions from this finding. There was no difference in the time to receive adjuvant therapy between the cohorts. We did not identify patient, disease, or treatment factors that were associated with new persistent use. The median time from surgery to completion of radiotherapy for the entire cohort was 13 weeks. These data suggest that judicious use of opioids results in a minimal risk of new persistent use and may aid in the delivery of adjuvant therapy within a favorable timeframe for patients with locally advanced OCSCC.

The data presented here contrast with outcomes reported in a recent publication of patients undergoing surgery with or without adjuvant therapy for OCSCC (12) in which 41% of the entire cohort required opioids more than 90 days after surgery. Of those patients, nearly 25% were new persistent users. Here we report only 13% of patients became new persistent users. These differences persisted despite more advanced primary tumors and regional disease and all patients receiving at least bimodality (surgery and adjuvant radiotherapy) and approximately 25% receiving trimodality therapy (surgery and adjuvant chemoradiotherapy). Smoking (18) and alcohol use (11), which have been demonstrated in prior studies to be associated with opioid use, showed minimal if no impact on persistent opioid use in either study. Given the small number of patients evaluated and found to be new persistent users, this may reflect a lack of power to identify a difference. The primary difference between the patient cohorts was the number of chronic users prior to surgery, which was associated with increased opioid prescription use in both studies. Hyperalgesia is a well described phenomenon for chronic opioid use (19), which is not accounted for in this study, but undoubtedly contributes to the clinical picture. It is unclear whether the increased opioid prescriptions for patients with previous use reflects this phenomenon, or use of opioids for other chronic pain conditions (19). These findings support cautious pain management approaches in patients with a history of chronic opioid use.

Previous data suggests that patients with OCSCC who are chronic users of opioids exhibit worse clinical outcomes (12). A possible rationale is that dysregulation of the immune system by opioids may enable tumors to escape immune-dependent tumoricidal activity (20). Other hypotheses suggest that opioids may result in tumor growth by activating the mu opioid receptors located on tumors, which can increase angiogenesis (21). There also is data to support worse outcomes with increasing doses of intra-operative opioid use (22, 23). Here we did not identify a difference in overall survival in patients that were non-persistent users compared to new persistent users. The differences in reports likely represent a lack of power and would require larger datasets to answer this question definitively.

Despite similar new persistent use of opioids identified in this study compared to others of approximately 10-15% (10, 11), strategies to reduce this risk should be pursued given their potential negative side-effects. As there is a neuropathic component to toxicities arising from treating OCSCC with surgery and radiotherapy, medications that block these signals may reduce pain and mitigate the need for opiates. Indeed, a recent randomized trial in patients with head and neck cancer receiving chemoradiotherapy demonstrated a reduction in opioid use with high-dose gabapentin compared to low dose gabapentin (24). However, pain continued to worsen over time in both treatment arms suggesting the need for further research in managing pain for patient with head and neck cancer receiving definitive treatment.

This study is limited by its sample size. Our ability to identify factors associated with new persistent use was limited given the small number of patients who required opioid prescriptions 3 months from the end of radiotherapy. Finally, we used opioid prescriptions as a surrogate use of opioid use. Without available records documenting a positive opioid drug test, the prescription surrogate was the best data available.

We demonstrate that persistent opioid use in patients with oral cavity squamous cell carcinoma undergoing curative intent surgery and adjuvant therapy is 13% which is similar to that reported by patients undergoing definitive treatment for various head and neck cancers (11). Caution should be taken when deciding about pain management approaches for patients with a recent history of opioid use given their increased propensity for use of these medications beyond cancer therapy. Future attempts at identifying novel agents beyond opioids should be pursued. However, given the strong association between the time of treatment and overall survival and the minimal risk of new persistent use and uncertain impact on overall survival, opioids should be used when clinically necessary.

ACKNOWLEDGMENTS

This work was supported in part by the NIH/NCI P30 CA014520-UW Comprehensive Cancer Center Grant and NIH P50 DE026787-UW Head and Neck SPORE Grant. Heather Geye for maintaining the Head and Neck cancer database. The authors declare that they have no conflict of interest. Informed consent was obtained from each individual participant involved in this study. This study was conducted in accordance with the 1964 Declaration of Helsinki and its subsequent amendments. There were no animals involved in this study.

REFERENCES

[1] Chaplin JM, Morton RP. A prospective, longitudinal study of pain in head and neck cancer patients. Head Neck 1999;21(6):531-7.

[2] Epstein JB, Stewart KH. Radiation therapy and pain in patients with head and neck cancer. Eur J Cancer B Oral Oncol 1993;29B(3):191-9.

[3] Keefe FJ, Manuel G, Brantley A, Crisson J. Pain in the head and neck cancer patient: Changes over treatment. Head Neck Surg 1986;8(3):169-76.

[4] Portenoy RK, Lesage P. Management of cancer pain. Lancet 1999;353(9165):1695-700.

[5] Saxena A, Gnanasekaran N, Andley M. An epidemiological study of prevalence of pain in head and neck cancers. Indian J Med Res.1995;102:28-33.

[6] Cuffari L, Tesseroli de Siqueira JT, Nemr K, Rapaport A. Pain complaint as the first symptom of oral cancer: a descriptive study. Oral Surg Oral Med Oral Pathol Oral Radiol Endod 2006;102(1):56-61.

[7] Frenette L. The acute pain service. Crit Care Clin 1999;15(1):143-50.

[8] Svensson I, Sjostrom B, Haljamae H. Influence of expectations and actual pain experiences on satisfaction with postoperative pain management. Eur J Pain 2001;5(2):125-33.

[9] Mandala M, Moro C, Labianca R, Cremonesi M, Barni S. Optimizing use of opiates in the management of cancer pain. Ther Clin Risk Manag 2006;2(4):447-53.

[10] Lee JS, Hu HM, Edelman AL, Brummett CM, Englesbe MJ, Waljee JF, et al. New persistent opioid use among patients with cancer after curative-intent surgery. J Clin Oncol 2017;35(36):4042-9.

[11] Smith WH, Luskin I, Resende Salgado L, Scarborough BM, Lin JY, Ozbek U, et al. Risk of prolonged opioid use among cancer patients undergoing curative intent radiation therapy for head and neck malignancies. Oral Onco. 2019;92:1-5.

[12] Pang J, Tringale KR, Tapia VJ, Moss WJ, May ME, Furnish T, et al. Chronic opioid use following surgery for oral Cavity cancer. JAMA Otolaryngol Head Neck Surg 2017;143(12):1187-94.

[13] Fujiwara RJ, Judson BL, Yarbrough WG, Husain Z, Mehra S. Treatment delays in oral cavity squamous cell carcinoma and association with survival. Head Neck 2017;39(4):639-46.

[14] Langendijk JA, de Jong MA, Leemans CR, de Bree R, Smeele LE, Doornaert P, et al. Postoperative radiotherapy in squamous cell carcinoma of the oral cavity: the importance of the overall treatment time. Int J Radiat Oncol Biol Phys 2003;57(3):693-700.

[15] Suwinski R, Sowa A, Rutkowski T, Wydmanski J, Tarnawski R, Maciejewski B. Time factor in postoperative radiotherapy: a multivariate locoregional control analysis in 868 patients. Int J Radiat Oncol Biol Phys 2003;56(2):399-412.

[16] Vikram B. Importance of the time interval between surgery and postoperative radiation therapy in the combined management of head & neck cancer. Int J Radiat Oncol Biol Phys 1979;5(10):1837-40.

[17] Goel AN, Frangos MI, Raghavan G, Lazaro SL, Tang B, Chhetri DK, et al. The impact of treatment package time on survival in surgically managed head and neck cancer in the United States. Oral Oncol 2019;88:39-48.

[18] Bastian LA, Driscoll MA, Heapy AA, Becker WC, Goulet JL, Kerns RD, et al. Cigarette smoking status and receipt of an opioid prescription among veterans of recent wars. Pain Med 2017;18(6):1089-97.

[19] Boudreau D, Von Korff M, Rutter CM, Saunders K, Ray GT, Sullivan MD, et al. Trends in long-term opioid therapy for chronic non-cancer pain. Pharmacoepidemiol Drug Saf 2009;18(12):1166-75.

[20] Boland JW, McWilliams K, Ahmedzai SH, Pockley AG. Effects of opioids on immunologic parameters that are relevant to anti-tumour immune potential in patients with cancer: a systematic literature review. Br J Cancer 2014;111(5):866-73.

[21] Singleton PA, Moss J, Karp DD, Atkins JT, Janku F. The mu opioid receptor: A new target for cancer therapy? Cancer 2015;121(16):2681-8.

[22] Cata JP, Keerty V, Keerty D, Feng L, Norman PH, Gottumukkala V, et al. A retrospective analysis of the effect of intraoperative opioid dose on cancer recurrence after non-small cell lung cancer resection. Cancer Med 2014;3(4):900-8.

[23] Cata JP, Zafereo M, Villarreal J, Unruh BD, Truong A, Truong DT, et al. Intraoperative opioids use for laryngeal squamous cell carcinoma surgery and recurrence: a retrospective study. J Clin Anesth 2015;27(8):672-9.

[24] Hermann GM, Iovoli AJ, Platek AJ, Wang C, Miller A, Attwood K, et al. A single-institution, randomized, pilot study evaluating the efficacy of gabapentin and methadone for patients undergoing chemoradiation for head and neck squamous cell cancer. Cancer 2020;126(7):1480-91.

In: Pain Management
Editors: J Merrick and M Morad
ISBN: 978-1-68507-493-7

Chapter 15

REGIONAL VERSUS GENERAL ANESTHESIA FOR PRIMARY TOTAL KNEE REPLACEMENT IN SAUDI ARABIA

Mariam Ahmad Alameri[1,*], PhD, Syed Azhar Syed Sulaimana[2], PhD, Abdullah Moh'd Talaat Ashour[3], MD, Ma'ad Faisal Al-Saati[4], MD and Maha Ali Al Draimlye, PhD

[1]Department of Biopharmaceutics and Clinical Pharmacy, Faculty of Pharmacy and Medical Sciences, Al-Ahliyya Amman University, Amman, Jordan
[2]Advance Medical and Dental Institute, Institut Perubatan dan Pergigian Termaju, Universiti Sains Malaysia, Bertam, Pulau Pinang, Malaysia
[3]Arthroplasty and Adult Reconstructive Surgery, Orthopaedics Department, Prince Sultan Military Medical City, Riyadh, Saudi Arabia

[*] ***Correspondence:*** Mariam Ahmad Alameri, B Pharm, MSc, Department of Biopharmaceutics and Clinical Pharmacy, Faculty of Pharmacy and Medical Sciences, Al-Ahliyya Amman University, Amman, 19328, Jordan. Email address: m_alamiri15@yahoo.com.

[4]King Abdullah bin Abdulaziz University Hospital,
Princess Nourah Bint Abdulrahman University, Riyadh, Saudi Arabia
[5]King Abduaziz Medical City Riyadh Ambulatory Care HCSC,
Riyadh, Saudi Arabia

ABSTRACT

The aim of this chapter is to compare morbidity and mortality for regional versus general anesthesia after primary total knee replacement (TKR). This is a prospective observational study that is done in two medical centers in Saudi Arabia. All patients who underwent primary TKR surgery in the included medical centers in a specific period were eligible for this study. A prospective data collection sheet was used to follow up each patient for 35 days post-surgery. 242 patients were participated in this study, 193 (79.8%) patients underwent regional anesthesia, and 49 (20.2%) underwent general anesthesia. There were statistically significant differences between the two groups in age, diseases, medications, Caprini score, length of hospital stay, length of surgery, day of achieving fully mobilization post operation, pulmonary embolism (PE) symptoms, sudden death, readmission, and medications' compliance evaluation. This study has proven that length of hospital stay, duration of surgery, days needed to achieve full mobilization post operation, PE symptoms, sudden death, and readmission are significantly higher in general anesthesia group.

LIST OF ABBREVIATIONS

VTE	venous thromboembolism
TKR	Total Knee Replacement
DVT	deep vein thrombosis
PE	pulmonary embolism
ICF	Informed consent form
PSMMC	Prince Sultan Military Medical City
KAAUH	King Abd Allah University Hospital
PNU	Princess Noura University
IRB	Institutional Review Board

BMI	Body Mass Index
HTN	Hypertension
DM	Diabetes Mellitus
IHD	Ischemic Heart Disease
US	United States
SSI	surgical site infection
PPI	Proton pump inhibitors
D1	day one
ACCP	American Collage of Chest Physicians

INTRODUCTION

In the last ten years, there were major changes in the delivery of orthopedic surgeries (1). The implementation of strategies such as day surgery admission and the use of spinal anesthesia resulted in a reduction in operating time also the proper analgesia which allows early mobilization and aggressive rehabilitation, resulting in a mean length of hospitalization of five days. These strategies contribute to decreasing the risk of death in the peri-operative period (2) and may reduce venous thromboembolism (VTE) since restricted movement and prolonged length of stay were common after joint replacement surgeries. According to the Clinical Practice Guidelines for Early Mobilization Hours after surgery, early ambulation is the most significant general measure to prevent postoperative complications, moreover, the postoperative benefits include a decrease in venous stasis, stimulation of circulation, prevention of VTE events, increases in muscle tone, coordination, and independence, and improved gastrointestinal, genitourinary and pulmonary functions (3). The aim of this study is to compare morbidity and mortality for regional versus general anesthesia after primary total knee replacement.

Our Study

This is a prospective observational study that is done in two medical centers in Saudi Arabia. Prince Sultan Military Medical City (PSMMC) located in Riyadh, which is considered as one of the most advanced medical centers in the Middle East with a capacity of about 1,200 beds, accredited by the International Joint Commission and King Abd Allah University Hospital (KAAUH), which is located in the southern area of Princess Noura University (PNU) Campus, a 300-bed teaching hospital serving PNU faculty.

All patients who underwent primary TKR surgery in the included medical centers between the period of October 2018 till July 2019 were eligible for this study. A prospective data collection sheet was used to follow up each patient for 35 days post-surgery. Type of anesthesia for each patient was dependent on surgeons' and anesthetists' experience. The study was approved by the Institutional Review Board (IRB) in both centers with Reference numbers (HP-01-R-079) and (H-01-R-059) for PSMMC and KAAUH respectively.

Inclusion criteria (patients who met all criteria will be included) were: Male or Female patients who are planned for elective TKR surgery (primary only), Agreed to sign the Informed consent form (ICF) and aged older than 18 years. Exclusion criteria were: Patients receiving anticoagulant for treatment, Patients with a history of DVT or PE, Patients with renal or hepatic failure, renal failure is defined as end-stage kidney disease (on dialysis); hepatic failure is defined as complete liver cirrhosis, pregnant woman, and revision surgeries.

Findings

242 patients were participated in this study, 193 (79.8%) patients underwent regional anesthesia, and 49 (20.2%) underwent general anesthesia. Table 1 shows Patients' demographic characteristics, the mean

age for all participants was 65.86 ± 8.96 and most of them were females 137 (56.6%). Body mass index (BMI) population mean was 32.46 ± 5.51. There were statistically significant differences between the two groups (regional/general anesthesia) in age, diseases (hypertension (HTN) and hypothyroidism), and medications (hypertension medications and antiplatelet). General anesthesia patients are significantly elder than regional anesthesia 68.51 ± 8.94 versus 65.19 ± 8.87 respectively. Two diseases out of 11 were significantly different with anesthesia type, these two diseases were; HTN and hypothyroidism. Among medications, there were two out 13 drugs that were significantly associated with anesthesia. These two drugs were anti-HTN and antiplatelet. Regional was higher 120 (49.6%) general 44 (18.2%) among HTN medication. Meanwhile, regional and general were equal 8 (3.3%), respectively, among antiplatelet. Surgical procedure, treatment, risk factors, and recovery measures during hospitalization were summarized in Table 2. There were significant differences according to anesthesia type in Caprini score, length of hospital stay, length of surgery, VTE prophylaxis postoperatively during hospitalization, the extended VTE prophylaxis, cost for extended VTE prophylaxis, day of achieving fully mobilization post operation. The mean ±SD Caprini score of regional was 7.74 ± 0.86 and for general was 8.22 ± 0.94. The mean ±SD of general and regional anesthesia for length of hospital stay were 6.35 ± 1.56 and 5.51 ± 1.21, respectively. Meanwhile, the mean ± SD of prescribed the general and regional anesthesia among length of surgery was 2.48 ± 0.79 and 2.07 ± 0.54, respectively. Among VTE prophylaxis postoperatively during hospitalization, Clexane 189 (78.1%) regionally and 46 (19.0%) generally was the highest prescribed VTE prophylaxis. Among extended VTE prophylaxis after discharge rivaroxaban 10 mg 118 (48.8%) regionally and 10 (4.1%) generally was the most prescribed drug. The mean ± SD cost for the extended VTE prophylaxis medications of general anesthesia $84.98 ± 35.21 was more than regional anesthesia $64.04 ± 42.45. The mean ± SD for days needed to achieve Fully mobilization post operation in general anesthesia group 4.88 ± 1.72 was higher than regional anesthesia 3.94 ±1.42.

Table 1. Comparing demographic and clinical data according to type of anesthesia

Demographics/Clinical data		Regional anesthesia 193 (79.8%)	General anesthesia 49 (20.2%)	All (N,%)	*p*
Age	Mean (SD)	65.19 (8.87)	68.51 (8.94)	65.86 (8.96)	0.020
Gender	Male (N,%)	87 (36.0%)	18 (7.4%)	105 (43.4%)	0.263
	Female (N,%)	106 (43.8%)	31 (12.8%)	137 (56.6%)	
BMI	Mean (SD)	32.72 (5.82)	31.43 (3.94)	32.46 (5.51)	0.146
Lifestyle*	Restricted (N,%)	91 (37.6%)	30 (12.4%)	121 (50.0%)	0.078
	Normally Active (N,%)	102 (42.1%)	19 (7.9%)	121 (50.0%)	
	Highly Active (N,%)	0 (0.0%)	0 (0.0%)	0 (0.0%)	
Diseases	Rheumatoid arthritis (RA) (N,%)	11 (4.5%)	0 (0.0%)	11 (4.5%)	0.087
	Dyslipidemia (N,%)	47 (19.4%)	15 (6.2%)	62 (25.6%)	0.370
	Osteoarthritis (N,%)	182 (75.2%)	49 (20.3%)	231 (95.5%)	0.087
	Benign prostatic hyperplasia (BPH) (N,%)	5 (2.1%)	3 (1.2%)	8 (3.3%)	0.217
	Asthma (N,%)	6 (2.5%)	3 (1.2%)	9 (3.7%)	0.319
	Diabetes mellitus (DM) (N,%)	117 (48.3%)	23 (9.6%)	140 (57.9%)	0.083
	Chronic kidney disease (CKD) (N,%)	1 (0.4%)	1 (0.4%)	2 (0.8%)	0.293
	Hypertension (HTN) (N,%)	121 (50.0%)	43 (17.8%)	164 (67.8%)	0.001
	Ischemic heart disease (IHD) (N,%)	19 (7.9%)	8 (3.3%)	27 (11.2%)	0.198
	Gout (N,%)	4 (1.7%)	0 (0.0%)	4 (1.7%)	0.310
	Hypothyroidism (N,%)	37 (15.3%)	16 (6.6%)	53 (21.9%)	0.042
	H2 blocker (Famotidine or Ranitidine)	33 (13.7%)	11 (4.5%)	44 (18.2%)	0.386
	Analgesic	193 (79.8%)	49 (20.2%)	242 (100.0%)	-
	A. B	193 (79.8%)	49 (20.2%)	242 (100.0%)	-
	VTE-Prophylaxis	193 (79.8%)	49 (20.2%)	242 (100.0%)	-

Demographics/Clinical data		**Regional anesthesia 193 (79.8%)**	**General anesthesia 49 (20.2%)**	**All (N,%)**	***p***
	DM-medication	117 (48.4%)	23 (9.5%)	140 (57.9%)	0.083
	HTN-medication	120 (49.6%)	44 (18.2%)	164 (67.8%)	0.000
	IHD-medication	19 (7.9%)	8 (3.3%)	27 (11.2%)	0.198
	Gout-medication	4 (1.7%)	0 (0.0%)	4 (1.7%)	0.310
	Proton pump inhibitors (PPIs)	133 (55.0%)	28 (11.5%)	161 (66.5%)	0.119
	Antiemetic	193 (79.8%)	49 (20.2%)	242 (100.0%)	-
	Levothyroxine	37 (15.3%)	14 (5.8%)	51 (21.1%)	0.150
	Statins	42 (17.4%)	15 (6.2%)	57 (23.6%)	0.192
	Antiplatelet	8 (3.3%)	8 (3.3%)	16 (6.6%)	0.002

AB = antibiotics, BMI = Body Mass Index, CKD = chronic kidney disease, DM = diabetes mellitus, HTN = Hypertension, IHD = ischemic heart disease, N = number or frequency of patients, OA = osteoarthritis, PPIs = Proton pump inhibitors, RA = rheumatoid arthritis, SD = standard deviation, TKR = total knee replacement, VTE = venous thromboembolism. To test the difference between continuous variables, compare means ANOVA test was used. Chi square was conducted to test discrete variables (frequencies). * Lifestyle: restricted means always sitting, normal means everyday life activity and highly active means exercising on daily basis.

Table 2. Surgical procedure, treatment, risk factors, and recovery measures during hospitalization

Demographics/Clinical data		Regional anesthesia 193 (79.8%)	General anesthesia 49 (20.2%)	All (N,%)	p
Caprini Score	Mean (SD)	7.74 (0.86)	8.22 (0.94)	7.83 (0.90)	0.001
Risk for bleeding	(N,%)	10 (4.1%)	1 (0.4%)	11 (4.5%)	0.346
Length of hospital stay	Mean (SD)	5.51 (1.21)	6.35 (1.56)	5.68 (1.32)	0.000
Type of metal implants	Cemented (N,%)	193 (79.8%)	49 (20.2%)	242 (100.0%)	-
	Cementless (N,%)	0 (0.0%)	0 (0.0%)	0 (0.0%)	
	Others (N,%)	0 (0.0%)	0 (0.0%)	0 (0.0%)	
Length of surgery	Mean (SD)	2.07 (0.54)	2.48 (0.79)	2.15 (0.62)	0.000
Pain Score	No pain (N,%)	0 (0.0%)	0 (0.0%)	0 (0.0%)	0.360
	Mild pain (N,%)	18 (7.5%)	2 (0.8%)	20 (8.3%)	
	Moderate pain (N,%)	43 (17.8%)	9 (3.7%)	52 (21.5%)	
	Sever pain (N,%)	132 (54.5%)	38 (15.7%)	170 (70.2%)	
Type of analgesia	No analgesia (N,%)	0 (0.0%)	0 (0.0%)	0 (0.0%)	0.277
	Non-opioid (N,%)	6 (2.5%)	0 (0.0%)	6 (2.5%)	
	Weak opioid (N,%)	34 (14.0%)	12 (5.0%)	46 (19.0%)	
	Strong opioid (N,%)	153 (63.2%)	37 (15.3%)	190 (78.5%)	
VTE- prophylaxis-pre-surgery during hospitalization	NON (N,%)	3 (1.2%)	0 (0.0%)	3 (1.2%)	0.068
	Clexane (N,%)	187 (77.3%)	46 (19.0%)	233 (96.3%)	
	UFH (N,%)	1 (0.4%)	3 (1.3%)	4 (1.7%)	
	Rivaroxaban (N,%)	1 (0.4%)	0 (0.0%)	1 (0.4%)	
	Aspirin (N,%)	1 (0.4%)	0 (0.0%)	1 (0.4%)	

Demographics/ Clinical data		**Regional anesthesia 193 (79.8%)**	**General anesthesia 49 (20.2%)**	**All (N,%)**	**p**
VTE prophylaxis-Post surgery during hospitalization	NON (N,%)	0 (0.0%)	0 (0.0%)	0 (0.0%)	0.041
	Clexane (N,%)	189 (78.1%)	46 (19.0%)	235 (97.1%)	
	UFH (N,%)	1 (0.4%)	3 (1.3%)	4 (1.7%)	
	Rivaroxaban (N,%)	2 (0.8%)	0 (0.0%)	2 (0.8%)	
	Aspirin (N,%)	1 (0.4%)	0 (0.0%)	1 (0.4%)	
After discharge VTE-Extended prophylaxis Analysis	Clexane 40 mg	49 (20.2%)	36 (14.9%)	85 (35.1%)	0.000
	Rivaroxaban 10 mg	118 (48.8%)	10 (4.1%)	128 (52.9%)	
	Aspirin 160 mg	26 (10.7%)	3 (1.3%)	29 (12.0%)	
Cost VTE Extended	Mean (SD)	64.04 (42.45)	84.98 (35.21)	68.28 (41.88)	0.002
Mobility within hours post operation (D0)	Yes (N,%)	3 (1.2%)	0 (0.0%)	3 (1.2%)	0.380
	No (N,%)	190 (78.6%)	49 (20.2%)	239 (98.8%)	
Fully mobilized no later than D1	Yes (N,%)	14 (5.8%)	3 (1.2%)	17 (7.0%)	0.782
	No (N,%)	179 (74.0%)	46 (19.0%)	225 (93.0%)	
Day for Start walking post operation	Mean (SD)	2.47 (1.10)	2.61 (1.01)	2.50 (1.08)	0.416
Day of achieving Fully mobilization post operation	Mean (SD)	3.94 (1.42)	4.88 (1.72)	4.13 (1.5)	0.000

D0 = same operation day, D1= after 24 hours post operation, SD = standard deviation, UFH = unfractionated heparin, VTE = venous thromboembolism. To test the difference between continuous variables, compare means ANOVA test was used. Chi square was conducted to test discrete variables (frequencies).

Table 3. Frequency of all complications post surgeries during follow up period

Demographics/Clinical data		Regional anesthesia 193 (79.8%)	General anesthesia 49 (20.2%)	All (N,%)	p
Pulmonary embolism symptoms	Yes (N,%)	0 (0.0%)	1 (0.4%)	1 (0.4%)	0.047
	No (N,%)	192 (79.7%)	48 (19.9%)	240 (99.6%)	
Sudden death	Yes (N,%)	0 (0.0%)	1 (0.4%)	1 (0.4%)	0.047
	No (N,%)	192 (79.7%)	48 (19.9%)	240 (99.6%)	
Deep vein Thrombosis symptoms	Yes (N,%)	11 (4.5%)	4 (1.7%)	15 (6.2%)	0.529
	No (N,%)	181 (75.1%)	45 (18.7%)	226 (93.8%)	
Confirm diagnosis (PE or DVT)	None (N,%)	181 (75.1%)	44 (18.3%)	225 (93.4%)	0.499
	Confirmed (N,%)	8 (3.3%)	4 (1.7%)	12 (5.0%)	
	Not confirmed (N,%)	3 (1.3%)	1 (0.4%)	4 (1.7%)	
Bleeding	No (N,%)	190 (78.8%)	49 (20.3%)	239 (99.2%)	0.473
	Yes, minor (N,%)	2 (0.8%)	0 (0.0%)	2 (0.8%)	
	Yes, major (N,%)	0 (0.0%)	0 (0.0%)	0 (0.0%)	
Surgical site Infection	Yes (N,%)	2 (0.8%)	0 (0.0%)	2 (0.8%)	0.473
	No (N,%)	190 (78.8%)	49 (20.3%)	239 (99.2%)	
Readmission	Yes (N,%)	2 (0.8%)	4 (1.7%)	6 (2.5%)	0.004
	No (N,%)	190 (78.8%)	45 (18.7%)	235 (97.5%)	
Did you take the VTE prophylactic medication as prescribed for you?	Yes (N,%)	191 (79.3%)	47 (19.5%)	238 (98.8%)	0.045
	No (N,%)	1 (0.4%)	2 (0.8%)	3 (1.2%)	
Tell its name, dose, and schedule	Can tell	142 (59.0%)	29 (12.0%)	171 (71.0%)	0.042
	Cannot tell	50 (20.7%)	20 (8.3%)	70 (29.0%)	
Duration for extended VTE Prophylaxis till day 35	Mean (SD)	20.24 (7.60)	18.61 (6.76)	19.91 (7.45)	0.172

DVT = Deep vein Thrombosis, PE = Pulmonary embolism, SD = standard deviation, VTE = venous thromboembolism. To test the difference between continuous variables, compare means ANOVA test was used. Chi square was conducted to test discrete variables (frequencies).

Frequency for all complications post surgeries during 35-days follow up period are shown in Table 3. There were significant differences according to anesthesia type in pulmonary embolism (PE) symptoms, sudden death, readmission, compliance evaluation question 1 and 2. General anesthesia 1 (0.4%) was only associated with PE symptoms in one patient, but the diagnosis could not be confirmed after using spiral computed tomographic scan of the chest. Similarly, General anesthesia 1 (0.4%) was only associated with sudden death. General anesthesia 4 (1.7%) was higher than regional anesthesia 2 (0.8%) among readmission cases. Regional anesthesia 191 (79.3%) and 142 (59.0%) was higher than general anesthesia 47 (19.7%) and 29 (12.0%) among compliance 1 and compliance 2, respectively.

CONCLUSION AND DISCUSSION

This study has proven that length of hospital stay, duration of surgery, and days needed to achieve full mobilization post operation, are significantly higher in general anesthesia group, which is supported by literature. The use of spinal anesthesia resulted in a reduction in operating time and may reduce VTE since restricted movement and prolonged length of stay were common after joint replacement surgeries (4). A meta-analysis study was done by Hu et al. (5) reveals that regional anesthesia seems to improve the outcomes of patients undergoing total hip or knee replacement, by reducing the operating time, the need for transfusion, and the incidence of thromboembolic disease; and this is shown in this study; there were significant differences between the two groups in PE symptoms, sudden death, readmission, and medications' compliance evaluation. General anesthesia group has recorded one death, one PE symptoms case, 4 readmission cases, and lower medications' compliance level. As a limitation for this study, this is an observational study, no randomization was used, instead the type of anesthesia was chosen according to surgeon experience and patients' specific conditions.

In this study, symptomatic VTE rate within 35 days post operation was 4.95% (12/242), which is within the international range for VTE incidence rate according to the reported literature, while symptomatic VTE rate during the first three months post orthopaedic surgery was within the range of 1.3% to 10% (6). In 2012, Murnaghan et al. stated that 12 from 2342 patients (0.6%) developed DVT, while 16 from 2342 (0.7%) patients developed PE (7). According to Loh et al. (2019), symptomatic DVT post TKR was 4.5% (8). Moreover, Murnaghan et al. (2012) concluded that all the early PE complications were seen in TKR surgeries, while late VTE events were seen in total hip replacement (THR) (7). According to Fuji et al. (2017), DVT, PE and bleeding incidence rate by surgery type was 1.3%, 0.2% and 1.0% for total knee replacement (9). In concordance with most of studies, only two cases of minor bleeding were seen in this study during follow-up period with a bleeding rate of 0.8% (2/242). In this study, majority of confirmed DVT cases, 12/242 (5%) were having regional anesthesia 8/193 (3.3%), while only 4/49 (1.7%) were having general anesthesia without a significant p-value. For major bleeding events, incidence rate was 0% while no cases of major bleeding were seen during the follow-up period, which is comparable to the reported literature for the bleeding rate post TKR where major bleeding events rate was only 0.04% (7). Regarding SSIs, the overall rate was 0.8% (2/242) for all patients, which was within the estimated international range. The overall rate of infection post orthopaedic surgeries was reported to be 0.55% up to 1.77% for primary surgeries, while for revision surgeries, it was 2.37% (9). Sudden death occurred for one case only with a rate of 0.4% (1/242); this case had a bilateral TKR under general anaesthesia. According to the National Centre for Health Statistics (NCHS), VTE was responsible for around one hundred thousand deaths each year in the United States and 25% of hospital sudden death cases was due to PE (10). Readmission rate for all patients was 2.5% (6/242) with four cases were having general anesthesia with a significant difference. This readmission rate was less than the rate reported by literature reported in literature, which was 4% for 30-day post TKR surgeries (11).

Conclusion

This is a prospective observational study that is done in two medical centers in Saudi Arabia; to prospectively compare morbidity and mortality for regional versus general anesthesia after primary total knee replacement. This study has proven that length of hospital stay, duration of surgery, days needed to achieve full mobilization post operation, PE symptoms, sudden death, and readmission, are significantly higher in general anesthesia group. Moreover, there were a significant difference between the two groups in medications' compliance evaluation with higher compliance in regional anesthesia group.

Acknowledgments

I gratefully acknowledge all surgeons at the surgical departments in both medical centers and a special thank for Dr Alwaleed Eid Alsubaie an associate's consultant orthopedic at Prince Sultan Military Medical City, and Dr Mohamed Ahmed Noaman ElRaei; an associate consultant orthopedic at King Abdullah bin Abdulaziz University Hospital for their cooperation and such attention. I greatly appreciate all the inpatients' nurses in both medical centers, especially, the inpatients' nurses at building 5 (ward 2) and building 2 from level 3 till level 7 at Prince Sultan Military Medical City, for their cooperation and guidance through the journey of this research. The study was approved by the Institutional Review Board (IRB) in both centres, first IRB was obtained from Research Ethics Committee, Scientific Research Center, Prince Sultan Military Medical City, Riyadh, Kingdom of Saudi Arabia-11149, with a reference number (HP-01-R-079). Second IRB was obtained from Institutional Review Board (IRB)OV 2018, Princess Nourah bin Abdulrahman University, Riyadh, Kingdom of Saudi Arabia, with a reference number (H-01-R-059). Consent forms were stacked to the survey (written consent forms were used). All authors confirm that the manuscript has been read and approved by all named authors. The order of authors listed in the manuscript has been approved by all named authors. The datasets used and analyzed during the current study are available from the corresponding author on reasonable request. This research did not receive any specific grant from any funding agencies in the public, commercial, or not-for-profit sectors. Conflict of interest: None to declare.

REFERENCES

[1] Jameson SS, Baker PN, Deehan DJ, Port A, Reed MR. Evidence-base for aspirin as venous thromboembolic prophylaxis following joint replacement. Bone Joint Res 2014;3(5):146-9.

[2] Kehlet H, Wilmore DW. Evidence-based surgical care and the evolution of fast-track surgery. Ann Surg 2008;248(2):189-98.

[3] Beverly A, Kaye AD, Ljungqvist O, Urman RD. Essential Elements of Multimodal Analgesia in Enhanced Recovery After Surgery (ERAS) Guidelines. Anesthesiol Clin 2017;35(2):e115-e143.

[4] Malviya A, Martin K, Harper I, Muller SD, Emmerson KP, Partington PF, Reed MR. Enhanced recovery program for hip and knee replacement reduces death rate. Acta Orthop 2011;82(5):577-81.

[5] Hu S, Zhang ZY, Hua YQ, Li J, Cai ZD. A comparison of regional and general anaesthesia for total replacement of the hip or knee: a meta-analysis. J Bone Joint Surg Br 2009;91(7):935-42.

[6] Goel R, Fleischman AN, Tan T, Sterbis E, Huang R, Higuera C, Parvizi J, Rothman RH. Venous thromboembolic prophylaxis after simultaneous bilateral total knee arthroplasty: aspirin *versus* warfarin. Bone Joint J 2018;100-B(1 Suppl A):68-75.

[7] Murnaghan J, Gollish J, Murnaghan D, Razmjou H, Donovan A, Bansal V. Thromboembolic and bleeding events following elective hip and knee arthroplasty using oral factor Xa inhibitor. Blood 2012;120(21):501.

[8] Loh JLM, Chan S, Wong KL, de Mel S, Yap ES. Chemoprophylaxis in addition to mechanical prophylaxis after total knee arthroplasty surgery does not reduce the incidence of venous thromboembolism. Thromb J 2019;17:9.

[9] Lecuire F, Gontier D, Carrere J, Giordano N, Rubini J, Basso M. Bilan de 10 ans de surveillance du taux d'infections du site opératoire dans un service d'orthopédie [Ten-year surveillance of nosocomial surgical site infections in an orthopedic surgery department]. Rev Chir Orthop Reparatrice Appar Mot 2003;89(6):479-86.

[10] National Center for Health Statistics (US). Health, United States, 2018. URL: https://pubmed.ncbi.nlm.nih.gov/31944640/.

[11] Urish KL, Qin Y, Li BY, Borza T, Sessine M, Kirk P, Hollenbeck BK, Helm JE, Lavieri MS, Skolarus TA, Jacobs BL. Predictors and Cost of Readmission in Total Knee Arthroplasty. J Arthroplasty 2018 Sep;33(9):2759-63.

In: Pain Management
Editors: J Merrick and M Morad
ISBN: 978-1-68507-493-7

Chapter 16

ASSOCIATION BETWEEN TYPE AND TYPE SPECIFIC INTENSITY OF CHRONIC PAIN WITH TIME-BASED DECISION MAKING

Marc Perlman**, MBA and John Huppertz, PhD
Albany Medical College, Albany, New York and Clarkson University, Schenectady, New York, United States of America

ABSTRACT

Compared to the general population, those suffering from chronic pain (CP) make aberrant decisions relating to time, which can influence their health behaviors and outcomes. By better understanding how the type and type-specific intensity of CP are associated with time preferences, providers can design interventions that allow patients to make improved health decisions. We conducted an online survey of U.S. adults to assess self-reported CP, present vs. future time preferences. Time preferences were evaluated via a Willingness-to-Accept instrument that used financial tradeoff scenarios to determine whether respondents were present-biased. Present bias refers to an individual's propensity to place

* ***Correspondence:*** Marc Perlman, MBA, Albany Medical College, 43 New Scotland Avenue, Albany, NY 12208, United States. Email: perlmam@amc.edu.

greater weight on present wellbeing over future wellbeing. Logistic regressions were performed to assess the relationship between present bias and CP type and type-specific intensity. Individuals who self-report CP were significantly more likely to be present-biased. In addition, total CP intensity, continuous CP intensity, and intermittent CP intensity positively predicted the likelihood of being present-biased. Ultimately, CP remains a multi-faceted construct that has substantial effects on decision-making. The disproportionately increased value that CP sufferers place on the present may influence their health behavior in a way that discounts future wellbeing.

INTRODUCTION

As a primary condition as well as a complication of other illnesses, chronic pain (CP) is a multidimensional construct that affects nearly all aspects of an individual's daily life. CP is defined as "pain that persists or recurs for more than three months" (1). This problem is particularly prevalent in the United States, prompting the Institute of Medicine to declare CP as a public health crisis (2). CP is associated with multiple diseases and chronic disorders, including heart failure, diabetes, cancer, depression, anxiety, sleep disorders, HIV, and multiple sclerosis (3), which are already difficult to manage. Medical professionals and CP patients alike have a deficit of knowledge about managing CP, complicating the treatment for these diseases even further (2). It is critical to explore how those with CP make decisions as these decisions have important implications for their health.

With upwards of 100 million people in the United States suffering from CP (4), this condition poses a tremendous burden on the US economy, resulting in costs estimated between $560 and $635 billion per year (2). In addition to the direct costs of providing CP diagnosis, management, and treatment, those with CP are more likely to have lower workplace productivity (5). Furthermore, CP is associated with atypical economic behavior as a result of numerous documented biases among those CP, such as risk-seeking behavior, delayed discounting, and recall bias (6-7). Previous literature has identified deviations in time-based decision making of CP patients, but no study has yet to relate the type and type-specific intensity of CP with time preference.

Time preferences

The behavioral economics literature on intertemporal decision-making is well-established, demonstrating the prevalence of biases that place higher values on immediate versus delayed rewards. Evidence suggests CP may impact one's intertemporal choices, decisions that involve multiple time periods (8). For example, the decision to exercise involves the short-term cost of time and energy in the current time period in exchange the long-term gain of improved health in a future time period. These intertemporal decisions are guided by an individual's valuation of both present and future.

A commonly used method of gauging an individual's intertemporal preferences is to calculate the discount factor. The discount factor revolves around the proposition that receiving a gain in the current time period is worth more than receiving that same gain in a future time period. For instance, the value received from $100 today may only be valued at $90 next month. The discount rate is a mathematical calculation that measures the anticipated value of future gains, so as to estimate the present value of those future gains. Thus, the time discount rate "express(es) the amount of future utility necessary to compensate an individual for waiting" (9).

Neoclassical economics would posit that an individual with a 10% monthly discount rate would be indifferent between receiving $100 today or $110 by deferring the payment to next month, and also indifferent between receiving $110 next month or $121 in two months. However, findings from the behavioral economics literature suggest that individuals tend to favor immediate gains disproportionately over delayed gains (10). This concept is known as present bias (the principal outcome measure of this study) and is characterized by the tendency to "give extra weight to well-being now over any future moment, but weigh all future moments equally (11). Individuals tend to choose the option that maximizes their utility in the present moment, but in situations when neither of the options provide utility in the present moment, people then temporally discount each outcome to identify the optimal course of action. The above example captures an individual who is not present-biased since they are indifferent to the two options that are of equal value when discounted. In contrast, an individual who is present-biased receives greater utility from receiving the reward in the present such that a $110 in one month may not be substantial enough for them to forgo the present reward of $100. However, for the tradeoff of $110 next month or $121 in two months, the individual is no longer considering a reward in the present, so the present bias is eliminated, and that individual would be indifferent to the two choices.

Time preferences are powerful predictors of health behaviors since they capture an individual's valuation of future and present wellbeing, and those with higher discount rates have been found to be at greater risk for obesity, smoking, and risky sexual activity, as well as lower likelihood of compliance with health recommendations (9). For example, temporal preferences have been linked to the likelihood of undergoing mammography screenings (12) and compliance with diabetes treatment (13). A better understanding of the time preferences of those with CP will allow for the design of more effective, timely, and appropriate interventions.

Objectives and hypothesis

Previous literature explored how CP affects intertemporal decision making and impulsiveness, but no study has deconstructed CP into type (continuous, intermittent, affective, and neuropathic) and type-specific intensity. By understanding the time preferences of those with CP, it is possible to better appreciate their decision-making process and help them make choices that maximize their long-term wellbeing.

This study explores whether the type and type-specific intensity of CP predict time preferences, or present bias (PB). In an online survey we compare a sample of those self-reporting CP with a random sample of adults in the U.S. The respondents' CP type and type-specific intensities comprise the independent variables, while the subjects' present bias (PB) comprises the dependent variable. Control variables included gender, age, race/ethnicity, education, income, and self-reported overall health. We hypothesize that in addition to previously established associations between general CP measures and PB, type-specific pain intensity measures would also uniquely predict PB.

OUR STUDY

Informed consent was obtained from each subject (see Appendix for procedures to obtain informed consent, survey, and opt-out). We used the SurveyMonkey Audience recruitment platform to recruit participants (>18-years old) to complete a 50-item survey. This platform accesses an online sample of pre-recruited respondents that were pre-screened for CP among other medical conditions. The participants receive compensation for completing surveys. We recruited two stratified samples: a random sample (RS; N=124) and a CP sample (N=154). For the CP sample, we added an additional screening question asking respondents to confirm they had CP, and respondents who reported not having or no longer having chronic pain (N=12) were disqualified from the study. While these two layers of screening were intended to confirm participants as having CP, the data are self-reported and there is no assurance that the participants necessarily meet the clinically accepted diagnostic criteria for CP. Of the RS, 39 individuals (31%) reported that they had CP, which is generally consistent the incidence of chronic pain among the U.S. population that is 18 years and older (2).

The research was approved by the Institutional Review Board of the authors' university.

Measures

Data on self-reported gender, age, race/ethnicity, education, income, and overall health status were collected. The item inquiring about overall health status is taken from the 2018 Behavioral Risk Factor Surveillance System Questionnaire (14) produced by the Centers for Disease Control (see appendix A).

The Short-Form McGill Pain Questionnaire (SF-MPQ) is a commonly used measure to test pain levels of CP patients across multiple dimensions (15). Recently updated to a second version, the SF-MPQ-2 assesses 22 descriptors of pain, and individuals rate each descriptor on a scale from 0 to 10, where 0 is 'none' where 10 is 'worst possible'. The SF-MPQ-2 is divided into four types:

- *Continuous CP*: pain that occurs constantly (e.g., throbbing, cramping, gnawing, aching, heavy, tender)
- *Intermittent CP*: pain that occurs at irregular intervals (e.g., shooting, stabbing, sharp, splitting, electric-shock, piercing)
- *Affective CP*: pain "characterized as eliciting complex emotional reactions" (e.g., tiring-exhausting, sickening, fearful, punishing-cruel) (16)
- *Neuropathic CP*: pain "caused by a lesion or disease of the somatosensory nervous system" (e.g., hot-burning, cold-freezing, pain caused by light touch, itching, tingling or "pins and needles," numbness) (17)

The SF-MPQ-2 measure is evaluated in terms of a person's total pain (a sum of each score) and pain intensity (total pain/number of descriptors chosen). In addition, these measures were calculated for each type and type-specific intensity of CP.

The minimum Willingness-to-Accept (WTA) instrument is a modified version of Meier & Sprenger's time preference measure (18). The WTA asks individuals to make six hypothetical payment decisions, asking them to determine a minimum dollar amount they would be willing to accept to forgo a payment of $500. In the first set of three decisions, individuals were asked to estimate the minimum payment needed to forgo receiving $500 right now, and in the second set of three decisions, they were asked to provide the minimum payment needed to forgo receiving $500 in six months. The first, second, and third question in each set proposes that an individual would have to wait one, two, or three additional months to receive their incremental payment.

Data analysis

Stata (version 16.1) was used to perform all data analysis. An alpha value of 0.05 was used as the threshold for statistical significance. Chi squared and two-tailed t-tests were used to compare differences between CP and RS groups.

For the SF-MPQ-2 analysis, several pain scores were derived based on methods outlined by Perlman and Raeburn (6). The analysis of the WTA time preference survey followed procedures described Meier & Sprenger (18), where Y represents the minimum dollar amount that the individual is willing to accept to wait, IDF is the monthly individual discount factor, and the $500 we used to create the scenarios is equivalent to the product of Y and IDF^d (where d is the delay period in months). IDF is calculated as:

$$\$500 = Y * IDF^{d}$$
$$IDF^{d} = 500/Y$$
$$IDF = (500/Y)^{1/d}$$

Each IDF is described as $IDF_{A,B}$, where A is the month at which the individual would receive the original payment (e.g., right now or in six months), and B is the month at which the individual would receive the delayed payment (1 month, 2 months, 3 months, 7 months, 8 months, or 9 months). Two distinct time frames are simulated through the comparison of $IDF_{0,1}$ with $IDF_{6,7}$, with the status quo scenario of receiving $500 right now ($IDF_{0,1}$) or receiving \$500 in 6-months ($IDF_{6,7}$). This instrument allows for the classification of a respondent as present- or future-bias by comparing $IDF_{0,1}$ and $IDF_{6,7}$. An individual will be classified as present-biased (PB1) if the value of $IDF_{6,7}$ divided by $IDF_{0,1}$ is greater than 1 and future-biased (FB) if this value is less than 1. The quotients of $IDF_{6,8}$, with $IDF_{0,2}$ (PB2) and $IDF_{6,9}$ with $IDF_{0,3}$ (PB3) were also calculated to assess robustness. PB1 is the outcome measure of focus for this study because $WTA_{0,1}$ and $WTA_{6,7}$ are thought to be the most easily visualized hypothetical decisions among the WTA items within their respective time periods.

Model specification

Logistic regressions were utilized to test the hypotheses. The general model specification is:

$$PB_i = \alpha + \beta_1 P_i + \beta_2 H_i + \boldsymbol{\gamma} X_i + \varepsilon_i$$

Where i is the individual respondent, PB_i is the present-bias categorical measure, P_i are the continuous pain measures, H_i is ordinal health measure and X_i are the categorical demographic controls.

FINDINGS

Due to the nature of the open-ended WTA instrument, some modifications and data cleansing were required. Specifically, all non-number responses were omitted or changed to numeric values. For example, "Nothing" was changed to numeric zero. Ambiguous responses such as "a lot" or "infinite" were excluded and assigned as missing values. Next, a value of 1.0 was added to all WTA-values to circumvent a divide-by-zero error inherent in the IDF calculation for respondents who answered '0'. In the two instances where respondents indicated they would not wait for any value, a placeholder of 1E10 was inserted. To account for outliers on the $WTA_{0,1}$ and the $WTA_{6,7}$ items, winsorization at the 95th percentile was performed, following Peters et al. WTA analysis (19). The 95th percentile was chosen since the large outliers present in about 5% of data.

Respondent characteristics

Characteristics of participants in the CP sample and the RS were similar, with the only significant demographic covariates being age and self-reported health, as shown in Table 1. Compared to the random sample (RS) the CP sample has a higher percentage of those older than 60 (49%) compared to the random sample's (28%) ($p=0.002$).Respondents in the CP sample present with worse self-reported health, with 41% reporting "poor or fair" health and only 14% reporting "good" health; in contrast, 22% of respondents in the RS reported "poor or fair" health and 42% reported "good" health ($p<0.001$). These expectations were consistent with epidemiological expectations, as the prevalence of chronic pain increases with age, and those with chronic pain are more likely to report worse overall health due to their pain (20).

There were no statistically significant differences in gender, race, income, or education between the RS and CP samples. With respect to self-reported pain, the CP sample had significantly higher scores across all pain measures (total pain, type-specific pain, total intensity, type-specific intensity, and each descriptor), as shown in Table 1. The samples did not significantly differ with respect to any of the Willingness-to-Accept items ($WTA_{0,1}$,$WTA_{0,2}$, $WTA_{0,3}$, $WTA_{6,7}$, $WTA_{6,8}$,$WTA_{6,9}$), the individual discount factor items ($IDF_{0,1}$, $IDF_{0,2}$, $IDF_{0,3}$, $IDF_{6,7}$, $IDF_{6,8}$, $IDF_{6,9}$), the bias variables (PB1, PB2, PB3, $IDF_{6,7}$ / $IDF_{0,1}$, $IDF_{6,8}$ / , $IDF_{0,2}$, or $IDF_{6,9}$ / $IDF_{0,3}$).

Table 1. Demographic comparison of chronic pain (CP) sample with random sample (RS)

Characteristic	CP Sample (% or mean)	CP SD	RS (% or Mean)	RS SD	Difference (p-value)
N (Number)	111	-	96		
Gender (% Female)	64	-	72	-	0.225
Age (%)		-			0.002
18-44	28	-	51	-	
44-60	23	-	21	-	
>60	49	-	28	-	
Race (% White)	87		77	-	0.051
Income (%)					
$0-$24,999	23	-	9	-	0.149
$25,000-$49,999	19	-	24	-	
$50,000-$74,999	20	-	21	-	
$75,000-$124,999	23	-	28	-	
>$125,0000	16	-	18	-	
Education (%)					<0.981
No HS, HS/GED, or Associate's Degree	24	-	22	-	
Vocational Degree or Some College	22	-	23	-	
Bachelor's Degree	29	-	30	-	
Graduate Degree	25	-	26	-	
Health (%)					<0.000
Poor or Fair	41	-	22	-	
Good	45	-	36	-	
Very Good or Excellent	14	-	42	-	
Total Pain	69.8	44.3	19.7	40.3	<0.000
Total NDC	13.6	5.5	3.6	6.3	<0.000
Total Intensity	5.0	1.9	1.7	2.7	<0.000
Total Continuous	22.4	13.4	6.2	12.2	<0.000
Continuous NDC	4.2	1.6	1.2	2.0	<0.000
Continuous Intensity	5.2	2.2	1.7	2.8	<0.000
Total Intermittent	19.5	15.3	6.0	13.9	<0.000
Intermittent NDC	3.7	1.9	1.0	1.8	<0.000
Intermittent Intensity	4.7	2.5	1.5	2.9	<0.000
Total Affective	13.2	10.0	3.4	7.7	<0.000
Affective NDC	2.4	1.4	0.6	1.2	<0.000
Affective Intensity	4.9	2.6	1.4	2.8	<0.000

Characteristic	CP Sample (% or mean)	CP SD	RS (% or Mean)	RS SD	Difference (p-value)
Total Neuropathic	14.7	12.7	4.0	8.7	<0.000
Neuropathic NDC	3.2	1.9	0.9	1.6	<0.000
Neuropathic Intensity	4.1	2.5	1.2	2.4	<0.000
PB1 (%)	92.8	-	88.5	-	0.291
PB2 (%)	94.6	-	93.8	-	0.795
PB3 (%)	94.6	-	95.8	-	0.679

Descriptive statistics of present bias

One-hundred and eighty-eight respondents (90.8%) were present biased, and 19 (9.2%) respondents were future-biased. The proportion of future-biased participants found in this study was consistent with the proportion of future-biased participants found in previous research (18).

Table 2. Comparison of those with present bias (PB) with those with future bias (FB)

Variable	PB (% or mean)	PB SD	FB (% or Mean)	FB SD	Difference (p-value)
N (Number)	188	-	19		
Gender (% Female)	69	-	53	-	0.143
Age (%)					0.661
18-44	38	-	47	-	
44-60	23	-	16	-	
>60	39	-	37	-	
Race (% White)	82		82	-	0.847
Income (%)					0.607
$0-$24,999	16	-	21	-	
$25,000-$49,999	21	-	26	-	
$50,000-$74,999	20	-	26	-	
$75,000-$124,999	26	-	21	-	
>$125,0000	18	-	5	-	
Education (%)					0.203
No HS, HS/GED, or Associate's Degree	22	-	32	-	
Vocational Degree or Some College	22	-	26	-	

Table 2. (Continued)

Variable	PB (% or mean)	PB SD	FB (% or Mean)	FB SD	Difference (p-value)
Bachelor's Degree	29	-	37	-	
Graduate Degree	28	-	5	-	
Health (%)					0.277
Poor or Fair	32	-	47	-	
Good	42	-	37	-	
Very Good or Excellent	27	-	16	-	
% with CP	71.3%	-	52.6%	-	0.0932
Total Pain	47.3	49.3	39.3	49.2	0.498
Total NDC	9.1	7.5	8.1	9.5	0.610
Total Intensity	3.5	2.8	2.6	2.8	0.181
Total Continuous	15.2	15.1	11.7	15.5	0.345
Continuous NDC	2.9	2.3	2.4	2.7	0.117
Continuous Intensity	3.7	3.0	2.5	2.8	0.380
Total Intermittent	13.6	16.3	10.4	14.4	0.411
Intermittent NDC	2.5	2.3	2.1	2.6	0.225
Intermittent Intensity	3.3	3.2	2.4	2.9	0.494
Total Affective	8.6	10.2	9.1	11.5	0.866
Affective NDC	1.6	1.5	1.6	1.9	0.376
Affective Intensity	3.4	3.2	2.7	3.1	0.991
Total Neuropathic	9.9	12.3	8.1	11.2	0.538
Neuropathic NDC	2.1	2.1	2.1	2.5	0.258
Neuropathic Intensity	2.9	2.8	2.1	2.9	0.892
$WTA_{0,1}$	$939.68	$552.50	$307.84	$252.41	<0.000
$WTA_{0,2}$	$1717.07	$1838.68	$430.47	$341.92	0.003
$WTA3_{0,3}$	$2502.03	$3109.11	$577.53	$536.17	0.008
$WTA4_{6,7}$	$2260.89	$3185.01	$937.84	$1189.49	0.074
$WTA5_{6,8}$	$2866.36	$4057.50	$1014.11	$1288.33	0.049
$WTA6_{6,9}$	$4185.97	$6972.18	$1215.47	$1552.18	0.066
$IDF1_{0,1}$	0.655	0.239	60.445	156.03	<0.000
$IDF2_{0,2}$	0.694	0.228	3.84	6.578	<0.000
$IDF3_{0,3}$	0.725	0.202	1.917	2.221	<0.000
$IDF4_{6,7}$	0.896	0.161	1.117	0.378	<0.000
$IDF5_{6,8}$	0.907	0.139	1.113	0.363	<0.000
$IDF6_{7,9}$	0.916	0.123	1.111	0.353	<0.000

Unadjusted univariate tests showed that present bias did not significantly differ by gender, race, age, education, income, or self-reported health status (see Table 2). Similarly, t-tests revealed that the majority of the pain measures and the bias variables (PB or the continuous value of $IDF_{6,7}/IDF_{0,1}$) were not significantly different across the present bias and the future bias groups. However, significant differences between the RS and CP samples were found on $WTA_{0,1}$, $WTA_{0,2}$, $WTA_{0,3}$, $WTA_{6,8}$, and all of the discount factors at the 0.05 level, and $WTA_{6,7}$ and $WTA_{6,9}$ were marginally significant at the 0.10 level.

Regression analysis

Preliminary regressions revealed that age was not significant in all models, so this covariate was omitted from the final models. In the final resulting model, there were 111 individuals in the RS and 96 individuals in the CP sample for whom there were complete data.

Table 3. Logistic regression between PB1 and amount and type of CP

Variables	(1)	(2)	(3)	(4)	(5)	(6)	(7)
Chronic Pain:	5.791***						
Yes	(1.595 - 21.03)						
Total Pain		1.011					
		(0.997 - 1.026)					
Total Continuous			1.053 (0.973 - 1.140)	1.042* (0.996 - 1.090)			
Total Intermittent			1.040* (0.995 - 1.088)		1.036* (0.997 - 1.078)		
Total Affective			0.935			1.025	
			(0.852 - 1.026)			(0.972 - 1.081)	
Total Neuropathic			0.984 (0.919 - 1.054)				1.040 (0.976 - 1.108)
Health Status: Good	2.959* (0.822 - 10.65)	2.592* (0.915 - 7.343)	1.981 (0.639 - 6.135)	2.488* (0.870 - 7.110)	2.455* (0.857 - 7.031)	2.162 (0.766 - 6.102)	2.441 (0.829 - 7.188)

Table 3. (Continued)

Variables	(1)	(2)	(3)	(4)	(5)	(6)	(7)
Health Status: Very Good or Excellent	6.404** (1.275 - 32.16)	4.207* (0.951 - 18.62)	3.682* (0.853 - 15.90)	4.376** (1.061 - 18.04)	3.949* (0.889 - 17.54)	3.324 (0.776 - 14.24)	3.669* (0.821 - 16.39)
Gender: Male	0.376*	0.412*	0.372*	0.420*	0.388*	0.419*	0.428*
	(0.139 - 1.016)	(0.152 - 1.116)	(0.126 - 1.098)	(0.153 - 1.149)	(0.143 - 1.052)	(0.154 - 1.139)	(0.157 - 1.164)
Education: Vocational Degree or Some College	1.037 (0.282 - 3.811)	1.003 (0.276 - 3.649)	0.883 (0.235 - 3.315)	0.970 (0.259 - 3.631)	1.000 (0.277 - 3.610)	1.021 (0.293 - 3.563)	1.014 (0.273 - 3.767)
Education: Bachelor's Degree	0.745 (0.223 - 2.487)	0.883 (0.272 - 2.868)	0.866 (0.258 - 2.910)	0.842 (0.258 - 2.751)	0.898 (0.274 - 2.945)	0.849 (0.264 - 2.732)	0.942 (0.290 - 3.058)
Education: Graduate Degree	5.039 (0.563 - 45.12)	7.423* (0.788 - 69.93)	7.006* (0.724 - 67.75)	7.031* (0.753 - 65.68)	7.765* (0.809 - 74.55)	6.867* (0.750 - 62.85)	7.054* (0.764 - 65.10)
Race: Non-white	1.904 (0.443 - 8.180)	1.508 (0.369 - 6.152)	1.549 (0.385 - 6.238)	1.547 (0.374 - 6.403)	1.550 (0.385 - 6.237)	1.405 (0.362 - 5.452)	1.366 (0.351 - 5.323)
Income: $25,000-$49,999	1.324 (0.283 - 6.187)	0.973 (0.200 - 4.733)	0.752 (0.130 - 4.366)	1.013 (0.204 - 5.019)	0.849 (0.183 - 3.946)	0.862 (0.197 - 3.766)	0.985 (0.197 - 4.929)
Income: $50,000-$74,999	1.010 (0.205 - 4.963)	0.845 (0.176 - 4.060)	0.628 (0.107 - 3.680)	0.841 (0.170 - 4.164)	0.751 (0.166 - 3.390)	0.736 (0.163 - 3.329)	0.869 (0.180 - 4.206)
Income: $75,000-$124,999	1.546 (0.292 - 8.188)	1.296 (0.246 - 6.832)	1.115 (0.195 - 6.357)	1.398 (0.262 - 7.455)	1.151 (0.229 - 5.787)	1.166 (0.238 - 5.717)	1.202 (0.235 - 6.143)
Income: >$125,000	5.777 (0.285 - 117.2)	3.743 (0.298 - 47.04)	2.901 (0.199 - 42.36)	3.908 (0.314 - 48.57)	3.368 (0.294 - 38.63)	3.316 (0.294 - 37.43)	3.361 (0.271 - 41.71)
Constant	0.205	2.712	4.353	2.548	3.340	4.587*	3.319
	(0.0103 - 4.077)	(0.473 - 15.54)	(0.655 - 28.91)	(0.474 - 13.70)	(0.728 - 15.33)	(0.993 - 21.20)	(0.547 - 20.14)
Observations	206	206	206	206	206	206	206
Psuedo-R2	0.1618	0.1295	0.1533	0.1359	0.1324	0.1081	0.1196

Robust 95% CI in parentheses.

*** p<0.01, ** p<0.05, * p<0.1.

Reference Categories: CP=No, Health=Poor or Fair, Gender=Female, Education=No H.S., H.S./GED, Associate's, Race=White, Income=<$24,999.

Table 3 presents the results from the logistic regressions with measures of total pain as the main independent variables. Self-reported CP was strongly associated with greater PB (AOR=5.791, 95% CI=1.595-21.030, $p<0.01$). Although total pain was not a significant predictor of PB, total continuous CP and total intermittent CP were marginally significant predictors of PB (AOR=1.042, 95% CI =0.996-1.090 $p<0.10$ and AOR=1.036, 95% CI=0.997-1.078, $p<0.10$ respectively).

PB and pain intensity

The logistic regressions involving PB and different measurements of pain intensity are found in Table 4. Total pain intensity marginally predicts PB (AOR=1.320, 95% CI=1.076-1.620, $p<0.10$). Both continuous CP intensity and intermittent CP intensity are positive predictors of PB (AOR=1.319, 95% CI=1.088-1.598, $p<0.01$ and AOR=1.289, 95% CI=1.076-1.544, $p<0.01$, respectively). Affective CP intensity and neuropathic CP intensity were only marginally significant positive predictors of PB (AOR=1.178, 95% CI=0.998-1.390, $p<0.10$; AOR=1.279, 95% CI=0.994 - 1.647, $p<0.10$).

Better health status is significantly associated with PB in many of the models. Compared to the reference group of "poor or fair" health, those with "good" health were significantly more present biased at the 0.05 level in two of the six models and marginally significant in four of the six models, with AORs ranging from 2.505 to 3.111. Similarly, compared to those with "poor or fair health," those with "very good or excellent" health were significantly more present biased in five of the six models and marginally significant in one of the six models, with AORs ranging from 4.197 to 5.663. With respect to gender, those who identify as male were marginally significantly less likely to be present-biased in five of the six models and significantly less likely to be present-biased in one of the six models, with AORs ranging between 0.337 and 0.421.

Table 4. Logistic regression between PB1 and CP intensity

Variables	(1)	(2)	(3)	(4)	(5)	(6)
Total Intensity	1.320*** (1.076 - 1.620)					
Continuous Intensity		1.300 (0.752 - 2.247)	1.319*** (1.088 - 1.598)			
Intermittent Intensity		1.171 (0.862 - 1.590)		1.289*** (1.076 - 1.544)		
Affective Intensity		0.831 (0.568 - 1.216)			1.178* (0.998 - 1.390)	
Neuropathic Intensity		1.058 (0.792 - 1.413)				1.279* (0.994 - 1.647)
Health Status: Good	3.016* (0.959 - 9.482)	2.988* (0.999 - 8.939)	2.807* (0.881 - 8.944)	3.029** (1.055 - 8.701)	2.505* (0.894 - 7.018)	3.111** (1.034 - 9.362)
Very Good or Excellent	5.648** (1.238 - 25.77)	5.663** (1.206 - 26.58)	5.485** (1.260 - 23.87)	5.431** (1.136 - 25.97)	4.197* (0.962 - 18.32)	4.835** (1.079 - 21.67)
Gender: Male	0.388*	0.337*	0.391*	0.347**	0.421*	0.408*
	(0.141 - 1.070)	(0.114 - 1.000)	(0.141 - 1.082)	(0.126 - 0.952)	(0.153 - 1.162)	(0.148 - 1.126)
Education: Vocational Degree or Some College	0.987 (0.261 - 3.736)	1.056 (0.254 - 4.385)	1.014 (0.261 - 3.935)	1.013 (0.266 - 3.849)	0.972 (0.268 - 3.534)	1.021 (0.269 - 3.881)
Education: Bachelor's Degree	0.880 (0.261 - 2.973)	0.933 (0.279 - 3.123)	0.883 (0.260 - 2.996)	0.942 (0.286 - 3.101)	0.886 (0.274 - 2.862)	1.026 (0.306 - 3.438)
Education: Graduate Degree	6.920* (0.691 - 69.32)	8.152* (0.704 - 94.46)	6.883* (0.706 - 67.11)	8.434* (0.818 - 86.99)	6.979* (0.709 - 68.68)	8.139* (0.834 - 79.40)
Race: Non-white	1.784	1.814	1.840	1.783	1.602	1.645
	(0.431 - 7.374)	(0.432 - 7.616)	(0.425 - 7.975)	(0.438 - 7.262)	(0.393 - 6.535)	(0.417 - 6.500)
Income: $25,000-$49,999	1.156 (0.232 - 5.764)	1.035 (0.181 - 5.919)	1.154 (0.224 - 5.944)	0.999 (0.211 - 4.729)	0.940 (0.215 - 4.102)	1.052 (0.209 - 5.292)

Variables	(1)	(2)	(3)	(4)	(5)	(6)
Income: $50,000-$74,999	0.955 (0.185 - 4.916)	0.854 (0.151 - 4.830)	0.924 (0.176 - 4.855)	0.867 (0.183 - 4.123)	0.789 (0.170 - 3.666)	0.800 (0.156 - 4.106)
Income: $75,000-$124,999	1.407 (0.261 - 7.595)	1.238 (0.203 - 7.535)	1.454 (0.261 - 8.096)	1.365 (0.249 - 7.494)	1.303 (0.255 - 6.657)	1.106 (0.219 - 5.581)
Income: >$125,000	4.612 (0.326 - 65.33)	4.426 (0.302 - 64.83)	4.638 (0.327 - 65.74)	3.999 (0.298 - 53.57)	3.271 (0.287 - 37.27)	3.341 (0.258 - 43.23)
Constant	1.535	1.702	1.566	1.894	2.888	2.128
	(0.305 - 7.738)	(0.317 - 9.149)	(0.322 - 7.624)	(0.396 - 9.065)	(0.618 - 13.51)	(0.376 - 12.03)
Observations	206	206	206	206	206	206
Pseudo R-squared	0.1530	0.1710	0.1597	0.1544	0.1258	0.1421

Robust 95% CI in parentheses.

*** $p<0.01$, ** $p<0.05$, * $p<0.1$ Reference Categories: CP=No, Health=Poor or Fair, Gender=Female, Education=No H.S., H.S./GED, Associate's, Race=White, Income=<$24,999.

Table 5. Comparison of WTA and IDF's between RS and CP sample

Characteristic	CP Sample (% or mean)	CP SD	RS (% or Mean)	RS SD	Difference (p-value)
$WTA_{0,1}$	$926.40	$631.74	$829.98	$467.25	0.220
$WTA_{0,2}$	$1784.76	$2037.01	$1384.17	$1444.30	0.101
$WTA_{0,3}$	$2637.41	$3424.48	$1964.59	$2435.32	0.110
$WTA_{6,7}$	$2510.39	$3595.97	$1710.55	$2288.00	0.062
$WTA_{6,8}$	$3131.12	$4481.86	$2193.65	$3099.91	0.087
$WTA_{6,9}$	$4754.15	$7967.98	$2941.10	$4738.40	0.053
$IDF1_{0,1}$	5.42	47.394	6.978	51.576	0.821
$IDF2_{0,2}$	0.932	2.050	1.041	2.286	0.719
$IDF3_{0,3}$	0.816	0.735	0.856	0.804	0.706
$IDF4_{6,7}$	0.902	0.176	0.933	0.225	0.274
$IDF5_{6,8}$	0.914	0.163	0.941	0.199	0.290
$IDF6_{7,9}$	0.923	0.153	0.947	0.181	0.306
$IDF_{6,7} / IDF_{0,1}$	1.528	.82	1.464	0.742	0.557
$IDF_{6,8} / IDF_{0,2}$	1.427	0.6	1.360	0.5	0.399
$IDF_{6,9} / IDF_{0,3}$	1.325	0.4	1.291	0.4	0.535

Time preference robustness assessment

In addition, these analyses were performed for PB2 and PB3 to assess for robustness as shown in Tables 6 through 9. PB2 is significantly positively predicted by the presence of CP (AOR=7.371, 95% CI=1.686-32.220, $p<0.01$) and intermittent CP intensity (AOR=1.325, 95%CI=1.051-1.570, $p<0.05$), as well as marginally significantly predicted by continuous CP intensity (AOR=1.267, 95%CI=0.997-1.160, $p<0.10$). PB3 was not significantly predicted by any of the pain measures. Overall, these analyses support that the primary results are moderately robust across time preference measures.

Table 6. Logistic regressions of PB2 and total CP

Variables	(1)	(2)	(3)	(4)	(5)	(6)	(7)
CP: Yes	7.371***						
	(1.686 - 32.22)						
Total Pain		1.012					
		(0.995 - 1.030)					
Total Continuous			1.027	1.040			
			(0.951 - 1.109)	(0.985 - 1.098)			
Total Intermittent			1.032		1.037		
			(0.975 - 1.092)		(0.988 - 1.088)		
Total Affective			0.942			1.018	
			(0.865 - 1.024)			(0.963 - 1.077)	
Total Neuropathic			1.029				1.064
			(0.930 - 1.139)				(0.966 - 1.173)
Health Status: Good	5.098*	3.827**	2.945	3.568*	3.503*	2.808	4.006**
	(0.882 - 29.45)	(1.001 - 14.64)	(0.739 - 11.74)	(0.905 - 14.07)	(0.901 - 13.62)	(0.764 - 10.32)	(1.000 - 16.04)

Variables	(1)	(2)	(3)	(4)	(5)	(6)	(7)
Health Status: Very Good or Excellent	19.58**	10.14**	8.093*	9.943**	9.282*	6.902*	9.709**
	(1.586 - 241.7)	(1.090 - 94.36)	(0.921 - 71.11)	(1.084 - 91.22)	(0.967 - 89.07)	(0.770 - 61.90)	(1.081 - 87.18)
Gender: Male	0.727	0.800	0.799	0.812	0.775	0.769	0.840
	(0.182 - 2.897)	(0.217 - 2.954)	(0.211 - 3.025)	(0.212 - 3.111)	(0.215 - 2.794)	(0.212 - 2.784)	(0.231 - 3.059)
Education: Vocational Degree or Some College	3.265	2.771	2.401	2.675	2.765	2.620	2.659
	(0.473 - 22.54)	(0.451 - 17.03)	(0.393 - 14.69)	(0.425 - 16.84)	(0.462 - 16.54)	(0.440 - 15.59)	(0.411 - 17.20)
Education: Bachelor's Degree	1.383	1.554	1.651	1.488	1.599	1.492	1.686
	(0.318 - 6.014)	(0.388 - 6.227)	(0.416 - 6.547)	(0.371 - 5.963)	(0.396 - 6.463)	(0.387 - 5.759)	(0.421 - 6.748)
Education: Graduate Degree	-	-	-	-	-	-	-
Race: Non-white	1.908	1.348	1.275	1.359	1.373	1.235	1.242
	(0.302 - 12.04)	(0.246 - 7.399)	(0.248 - 6.569)	(0.252 - 7.332)	(0.258 - 7.299)	(0.248 - 6.140)	(0.227 - 6.800)
Income: \$25,000-\$49,999	1.570	1.077	0.885	1.073	0.910	0.901	1.274
	(0.233 - 10.58)	(0.135 - 8.565)	(0.0857 - 9.145)	(0.141 - 8.180)	(0.131 - 6.318)	(0.146 - 5.556)	(0.132 - 12.31)
Income: \$50,000-\$74,999	0.569	0.501	0.435	0.474	0.445	0.430	0.594
	(0.0869 - 3.726)	(0.0781 - 3.208)	(0.0533 - 3.548)	(0.0754 - 2.978)	(0.0754 - 2.629)	(0.0744 - 2.490)	(0.0882 - 4.003)
Income \$75,000-\$124,999	1.527	1.356	1.131	1.393	1.213	1.163	1.342
	(0.198 - 11.80)	(0.169 - 10.90)	(0.136 - 9.394)	(0.175 - 11.06)	(0.160 - 9.205)	(0.159 - 8.527)	(0.176 - 10.24)
Income: >\$125,999	-	-	-	-	-	-	-
Constant	0.0846	1.793	2.634	1.886	2.288	3.801	1.598
	(0.00349 - 2.050)	(0.224 - 14.37)	(0.296 - 23.46)	(0.260 - 13.70)	(0.387 - 13.51)	(0.725 - 19.94)	(0.190 - 13.46)
Observations	134	134	134	134	134	134	134

Robust 95%CI in parentheses.

*** p<0.01, ** p<0.05, * p<0.1 Reference Categories: CP=No, Health=Poor or Fair, Gender=Female, Education=No H.S., H.S./GED, Associate's, Race=White, Income=<\$24,999.

Table 7. Logistic regressions of PB2 and CP intensity

Variables	**(1)**	**(2)**	**(3)**	**(4)**	**(5)**	**(6)**
Total Intensity	1.280*					
	(0.988 - 1.657)					
Continuous Intensity		0.972	1.267*			
		(0.492 - 1.921)	(0.997 - 1.610)			
Intermittent Intensity		1.486		1.325**		
		(0.926 - 2.386)		(1.051 - 1.670)		
Affective Intensity		0.824			1.163	
		(0.519 - 1.307)			(0.952 - 1.421)	
Neuropathic Intensity		1.135				1.326
		(0.754 - 1.708)				(0.927 - 1.897)
Health Status: Good	4.215*	5.046**	3.910*	4.765**	3.522*	4.789**
	(0.856 - 20.74)	(1.313 - 19.39)	(0.809 - 18.91)	(1.159 - 19.60)	(0.924 - 13.43)	(1.128 - 20.34)
Health Status: Very Good or Excellent	12.77**	15.39**	12.17**	14.87**	9.403*	12.91**
	(1.185 - 137.8)	(1.416 - 167.2)	(1.107 - 133.8)	(1.279 - 173.0)	(0.969 - 91.21)	(1.309 - 127.3)
Gender: Male	0.715	0.578	0.714	0.636	0.758	0.750
	(0.188 - 2.718)	(0.135 - 2.481)	(0.184 - 2.769)	(0.163 - 2.483)	(0.202 - 2.848)	(0.187 - 3.002)
Education: Vocational Degree or Some College	2.874	3.348	2.913	3.122	2.632	2.879
	(0.448 - 18.46)	(0.494 - 22.70)	(0.435 - 19.49)	(0.476 - 20.47)	(0.428 - 16.19)	(0.445 - 18.61)
Education: Bachelor's Degree	1.559	1.973	1.544	1.708	1.524	1.870
	(0.380 - 6.392)	(0.524 - 7.429)	(0.370 - 6.438)	(0.420 - 6.942)	(0.389 - 5.964)	(0.451 - 7.749)
Education: Graduate Degree	-	-	-	-	-	-
Race: Non-white	1.614	1.737	1.629	1.697	1.430	1.635
	(0.291 - 8.944)	(0.319 - 9.445)	(0.288 - 9.216)	(0.299 - 9.632)	(0.258 - 7.925)	(0.303 - 8.829)

Variables	(1)	(2)	(3)	(4)	(5)	(6)
Income:	1.152	0.962	1.114	1.046	0.980	1.164
$25,000-$49,999	(0.161 - 8.258)	(0.111 - 8.345)	(0.157 - 7.892)	(0.142 - 7.687)	(0.155 - 6.204)	(0.137 - 9.903)
Income:	0.520	0.424	0.493	0.489	0.468	0.461
$50,000-$74,999	(0.0788 - 3.428)	(0.0575 - 3.124)	(0.0764 - 3.180)	(0.0784 - 3.053)	(0.0762 - 2.868)	(0.0608 - 3.504)
Income	1.338	1.073	1.372	1.390	1.309	1.082
$75,000-$124,999	(0.174 - 10.27)	(0.125 - 9.221)	(0.171 - 11.02)	(0.154 - 12.59)	(0.169 - 10.16)	(0.146 - 8.015)
Income: >$125,999	-	-	-	-	-	-
Constant	1.287	1.284	1.393	1.179	2.240	1.309
	(0.190 - 8.711)	(0.162 - 10.18)	(0.223 - 8.714)	(0.180 - 7.713)	(0.376 - 13.36)	(0.148 - 11.57)
Observations	134	134	134	134	134	134

Robust 95% CI in parentheses.

*** $p<0.01$, ** $p<0.05$, * $p<0.1$ Reference Categories: CP=No, Health=Poor or Fair, Gender=Female, Education=No H.S., H.S./GED, Associate's, Race=White, Income=<$24,999.

Table 8. Logistic regressions of PB3 and total CP

Variables	(1)	(2)	(3)	(4)	(5)	(6)	(7)
CP: Yes	4.355						
	(0.473 - 40.09)						
Total Pain		1.007					
		(0.991 - 1.023)					
Total			1.048	1.031			
Continuous			(0.967 - 1.135)	(0.976 - 1.089)			
Total			1.001		1.015		
Intermittent			(0.933 - 1.074)		(0.974 - 1.057)		
Total			0.929			0.991	
Affective			(0.836 - 1.033)			(0.927 - 1.060)	
Total			1.033				1.050
Neuropathic			(0.939 - 1.136)				(0.951 - 1.160)
Health	11.32**	9.065**	6.700**	9.781**	8.097**	6.034**	10.53**
Status: Good	(1.008 - 127.0)	(1.573 - 52.25)	(1.254 - 35.79)	(1.528 - 62.60)	(1.358 - 48.28)	(1.234 - 29.50)	(1.615 - 68.60)

Table 8. (Continued)

Variables	(1)	(2)	(3)	(4)	(5)	(6)	(7)
Health Status: Very Good or Excellent	-	-	-	-	-	-	-
Gender: Male	0.266*	0.290	0.298	0.294	0.285*	0.283*	0.303
	(0.0569 - 1.242)	(0.0659 - 1.279)	(0.0579 - 1.538)	(0.0652 - 1.325)	(0.0656 - 1.240)	(0.0640 - 1.248)	(0.0668 - 1.371)
Education: Vocational Degree or Some College	3.448	2.838	2.178	2.946	2.688	2.475	2.744
	(0.491 - 24.24)	(0.457 - 17.62)	(0.305 - 15.57)	(0.451 - 19.25)	(0.428 - 16.88)	(0.425 - 14.40)	(0.392 - 19.23)
Education: Bachelor's Degree	1.361	1.391	1.481	1.333	1.369	1.291	1.592
	(0.241 - 7.678)	(0.271 - 7.140)	(0.306 - 7.165)	(0.256 - 6.934)	(0.264 - 7.094)	(0.246 - 6.768)	(0.314 - 8.061)
Education: Graduate Degree	-	-	-	-	-	-	-
Race: Non-white	3.706	2.637	2.343	2.769	2.582	2.305	2.600
	(0.504 - 27.23)	(0.321 - 21.65)	(0.303 - 18.09)	(0.338 - 22.67)	(0.309 - 21.59)	(0.275 - 19.35)	(0.310 - 21.82)
Income: \$25,000-\$49,999	1.279	0.962	1.019	0.990	0.878	0.904	1.236
	(0.162 - 10.08)	(0.0988 - 9.362)	(0.0549 - 18.92)	(0.0963 - 10.18)	(0.103 - 7.481)	(0.117 - 7.003)	(0.0812 - 18.82)
Income: \$50,000-\$74,999	0.297	0.292	0.288	0.274	0.278	0.278	0.372
	(0.0386 - 2.286)	(0.0389 - 2.193)	(0.0264 - 3.153)	(0.0362 - 2.071)	(0.0397 - 1.947)	(0.0434 - 1.780)	(0.0400 - 3.448)
Income \$75,000-\$124,999	1.970	1.723	1.538	1.835	1.635	1.626	1.705
	(0.104 - 37.21)	(0.104 - 28.64)	(0.0912 - 25.95)	(0.104 - 32.38)	(0.107 - 24.99)	(0.101 - 26.16)	(0.104 - 27.96)
Income: >\$125,999	-	-	-	-	-	-	-
Constant	0.302	3.373	4.447	2.820	4.380	7.549**	2.267
	(0.00353 - 25.91)	(0.341 - 33.38)	(0.303 - 65.26)	(0.303 - 26.26)	(0.583 - 32.89)	(1.038 - 54.90)	(0.171 - 30.01)
Observations	104	104	104	104	104	104	104

Robust 95 CI in parentheses.

*** p<0.01, ** p<0.05, * p<0.1 Reference Categories: CP=No, Health=Poor or Fair, Gender=Female, Education=No H.S., H.S./GED, Associate's, Race=White, Income=<\$24,999.

Table 9. Logistic regressions of PB3 and CP intensity

Variables	(1)	(2)	(3)	(4)	(5)	(6)
Total Intensity	1.020					
	(0.714 - 1.457)					
Continuous Intensity		1.028	1.101			
		(0.371 - 2.852)	(0.801 - 1.513)			
Intermittent Intensity		1.464		1.125		
		(0.879 - 2.438)		(0.855 - 1.480)		
Affective Intensity		0.716			0.998	
		(0.382 - 1.344)			(0.757 - 1.316)	
Neuropathic Intensity		0.989				1.101
		(0.735 - 1.331)				(0.813 - 1.492)
Health Status: Good	7.003*	7.762**	8.483**	9.393**	6.617**	8.806**
	(0.882 - 55.61)	(1.521 - 39.62)	(1.027 - 70.08)	(1.667 - 52.95)	(1.333 - 32.84)	(1.321 - 58.70)
Health Status: Very Good or Excellent	-	-	-	-	-	-
Gender: Male	0.282*	0.187**	0.271*	0.252*	0.284*	0.278*
	(0.0634 - 1.255)	(0.0360 - 0.969)	(0.0605 - 1.214)	(0.0587 - 1.085)	(0.0647 - 1.247)	(0.0638 - 1.208)
Education: Vocational Degree or Some College	2.618	3.049	2.913	2.874	2.577	2.735
	(0.415 - 16.52)	(0.393 - 23.67)	(0.421 - 20.15)	(0.447 - 18.49)	(0.421 - 15.78)	(0.428 - 17.48)
Education: Bachelor's Degree	1.327	1.572	1.388	1.445	1.302	1.529
	(0.222 - 7.951)	(0.290 - 8.530)	(0.249 - 7.741)	(0.273 - 7.661)	(0.248 - 6.843)	(0.258 - 9.055)
Education: Graduate Degree	-	-	-	-	-	-
Race: Non-white	2.437	2.618	2.798	2.901	2.348	2.836
	(0.302 - 19.70)	(0.341 - 20.09)	(0.349 - 22.44)	(0.368 - 22.85)	(0.288 - 19.14)	(0.324 - 24.81)
Income: \$25,000-\$49,999	0.923	0.752	0.970	0.938	0.911	0.997
	(0.119 - 7.184)	(0.0759 - 7.439)	(0.115 - 8.214)	(0.108 - 8.176)	(0.115 - 7.224)	(0.108 - 9.201)

Table 9. (Continued)

Variables	(1)	(2)	(3)	(4)	(5)	(6)
Income:	0.282	0.280	0.281	0.288	0.281	0.273
\$50,000- \$74,999	(0.0430 - 1.850)	(0.0357 - 2.203)	(0.0395 - 2.006)	(0.0399 - 2.077)	(0.0431 - 1.826)	(0.0401 - 1.858)
Income	1.668	1.424	1.734	1.764	1.655	1.546
\$75,000- \$124,999	(0.107 - 25.98)	(0.0633 - 32.01)	(0.105 - 28.51)	(0.0965 - 32.27)	(0.0951 - 28.79)	(0.102 - 23.40)
Income: >\$125,999	-	-	-	-	-	-
Constant	5.586	5.337	3.559	3.212	6.386	3.735
	(0.391 - 79.76)	(0.406 - 70.14)	(0.307 - 41.19)	(0.300 - 34.36)	(0.615 - 66.28)	(0.297 - 46.93)
Observations	104	104	104	104	104	104

Robust 95 CI in parentheses.

*** p<0.01, ** p<0.05, * p<0.1 Reference Categories: CP=No, Health=Poor or Fair, Gender=Female, Education=No H.S., H.S./GED, Associate's, Race=White, Income=<\$24,999.

Table 10. Logistic regressions of PB1 and individual pain descriptors

Pain Descriptors	(1)	(2)	(3)	(4)	(5)
Throbbing	1.053	0.854			
	(0.742 - 1.495)	(0.649 - 1.124)			
Cramping	0.854	0.976			
	(0.565 - 1.289)	(0.790 - 1.207)			
Gnawing	1.165	1.143			
	(0.743 - 1.826)	(0.879 - 1.487)			
Aching	1.307	1.359**			
	(0.949 - 1.800)	(1.074 - 1.720)			
Heavy	0.606**	1.039			
	(0.412 - 0.891)	(0.862 - 1.252)			
Tender	1.249	0.846			
	(0.870 - 1.792)	(0.688 - 1.040)			
Shooting	1.136		1.278*		
	(0.812 - 1.587)		(0.989 - 1.653)		

Pain Descriptors	(1)	(2)	(3)	(4)	(5)
Stabbing	0.690*		1.011		
	(0.459 - 1.038)		(0.770 - 1.326)		
Sharp	1.730***		1.030		
	(1.158 - 2.585)		(0.822 - 1.290)		
Splitting	0.473***		0.854		
	(0.306 - 0.729)		(0.676 - 1.079)		
Electric-shock	0.897		0.951		
	(0.573 - 1.406)		(0.793 - 1.141)		
Piercing	3.353***		1.118		
	(1.936 - 5.810)		(0.897 - 1.394)		
Tiring-exhausting	0.911			1.112	
	(0.591 - 1.405)			(0.897 - 1.377)	
Sickening	1.411			1.027	
	(0.719 - 2.767)			(0.827 - 1.277)	
Fearful	0.669			0.806**	
	(0.366 - 1.220)			(0.653 - 0.996)	
Punishing-cruel	0.831			1.106	
	(0.524 - 1.317)			(0.908 - 1.348)	
Hot-burning	1.096				1.190*
	(0.804 - 1.493)				(0.990 - 1.430)
Cold-freezing	1.159				0.979
	(0.664 - 2.022)				(0.570 - 1.681)
Pain caused by light touch	0.517***				0.827
	(0.340 - 0.787)				(0.647 - 1.057)
Itching	1.442**				1.208
	(1.029 - 2.021)				(0.940 - 1.551)

Table 10. (Continued)

Pain Descriptors	(1)	(2)	(3)	(4)	(5)
Tingling or 'pins and needles'	1.444*				1.295**
	(0.990 - 2.106)				(1.056 - 1.588)
Numbness	0.652**				0.808*
	(0.458 - 0.930)				(0.649 - 1.007)
Gender: Male	0.195**	0.285**	0.436	0.340*	0.378*
	(0.0499 - 0.765)	(0.0863 - 0.943)	(0.153 - 1.242)	(0.110 - 1.050)	(0.129 - 1.108)
Health Status: Good	5.513*	2.851*	2.474*	2.768*	3.187*
	(0.758 - 40.08)	(0.882 - 9.217)	(0.854 - 7.168)	(0.906 - 8.453)	(0.871 - 11.66)
Health Status: Very Good or Excellent	10.51**	4.719**	4.354*	4.274*	3.707*
	(1.211 - 91.17)	(1.058 - 21.05)	(0.952 - 19.91)	(0.945 - 19.34)	(0.849 - 16.18)
Education: Vocational Degree or Some College	0.405	0.683	1.028	0.729	0.802
	(0.0560 - 2.934)	(0.145 - 3.222)	(0.283 - 3.738)	(0.200 - 2.648)	(0.210 - 3.057)
Education: Bachelor's Degree	0.905	0.697	1.121	0.756	0.944
	(0.131 - 6.271)	(0.170 - 2.860)	(0.325 - 3.861)	(0.235 - 2.437)	(0.263 - 3.387)
Education: Graduate Degree	6.575	4.454	8.941*	5.874	6.115
	(0.126 - 344.2)	(0.389 - 51.05)	(0.932 - 85.82)	(0.566 - 60.99)	(0.628 - 59.53)
Race: Non-white	6.064*	1.872	1.787	1.701	1.837
	(0.828 - 44.43)	(0.483 - 7.253)	(0.454 - 7.029)	(0.440 - 6.569)	(0.506 - 6.671)
Income: $25,000-$49,999	0.118**	0.577	1.096	0.717	0.953
	(0.0193 - 0.727)	(0.119 - 2.800)	(0.237 - 5.079)	(0.162 - 3.174)	(0.145 - 6.243)
Income: $50,000-$74,999	0.114**	0.483	0.731	0.476	1.090
	(0.0147 - 0.883)	(0.0945 - 2.471)	(0.148 - 3.609)	(0.0965 - 2.351)	(0.206 - 5.782)
Income: $75,000-$124,999	0.106**	0.598	1.249	0.942	1.022
	(0.0132 - 0.852)	(0.107 - 3.350)	(0.221 - 7.059)	(0.172 - 5.158)	(0.177 - 5.882)
Income: >$125,000	1.098	2.360	3.356	2.571	4.951
	(0.0651 - 18.51)	(0.195 - 28.51)	(0.270 - 41.77)	(0.196 - 33.77)	(0.305 - 80.29)
Constant	11.69**	6.056*	2.197	5.291*	2.843
	(1.361 - 100.4)	(0.993 - 36.92)	(0.395 - 12.23)	(0.869 - 32.23)	(0.342 - 23.63)

Pain Descriptors	(1)	(2)	(3)	(4)	(5)
Observations	187	195	200	203	198
Pseudo R-squared	0.3529	0.1914	0.1558	0.1361	0.1757

Robust 95 CI in parentheses.

*** p<0.01, ** p<0.05, * p<0.1.

Reference Categories: CP=No, Health=Poor or Fair, Gender=Female, Education=No H.S., H.S./GED, Associate's, Race=White, Income=<$24,999.

DISCUSSION

Overall, the data support that CP positively predicts PB, suggesting that those with CP are more likely to prefer small gains sooner rather than larger gains later. The condition of CP increases the odds that individual will have PB by almost six times (see Table 3). This finding is generally consistent with previous research findings that show those with CP tend to disproportionately value present gains over future gains (7). However, ours is the first study to examine the role of CP intensity and type-specific intensity on PB. This study finds a significant association between type-specific intensity and time preferences, where CP intensity, continuous CP intensity, and intermittent CP intensity positively predicted the likelihood of being present-biased.

The results support the hypothesis that type-specific CP intensity is significantly related to PB. Although the total quantity of pain (and type-specific pain) was not significantly associated with present bias, pain intensity was a significant predictor. Recall that pain intensity is defined as the total quantity of pain divided by the number of the pain descriptors chosen. This finding suggests that the severity of the total and type-specific pain is more impactful on intertemporal decision-making than the quantity of pain. In other words, if a patient with CP describes their pain with a large number of descriptors, this may not necessarily lead to present bias. It can be extrapolated that a patient with one CP descriptor (e.g., piercing) that is interpreted as the worst possible (i.e., 10/10) is more present-biased than individual with five CP descriptors that are ranked at 2/10 each, despite reporting the same amount of experienced total pain.

Type-specific intensity measures also emerged in our analyses, as continuous and intermittent CP intensity were both significant predictors of PB. To our knowledge, this is the first study to assess the relationship between the type and type-specific intensities of CP with time preference. A potential explanation for why continuous and intermittent CP intensity were significant CP predictors of PB can draw upon domain-dependence. Both continuous and intermittent CP are types of CP that are functions of time. Continuous CP is constant, and intermittent CP arises at varying intervals. Temporal types of pain lead to temporal biases (i.e., present bias), suggesting domain-dependence between CP intensity and cognitive bias.

This study serves to further the work by Perlman and Raeburn (6), which evaluated the relationship between the type and type-specific intensity of CP on risk preferences (6). The principal outcome of that study was that neuropathic intensity significantly predicted an individual's willingness to take risks with respect to their health. Neuropathic CP is associated with a worse quality of life than other types of CP, including more "frequent and severe sleep disturbances, anxiety, and depression" (21). Such a significant symptom burden may negatively influence one's ability to weigh the benefits and drawbacks of different decisions, explaining their increased willingness to take risks with respect to their health. It was surprising to discover in this study that neuropathic intensity only predicted PB at the 0.10 level. With a larger sample size, this relationship may be affirmed.

Another key finding of previous work was the concept of domain-dependence with respect to the category of stressor and the category of decision. CP (a health stressor) was found to predict an individuals' health-related risk preferences while lower income (a financial stressor) significantly predicts an individual's financial-related risks. This domain-dependence provides a rationale for the current study's finding that continuous and intermittent CP, both time-related types of CP, are related to PB, a time-related bias.

The novel contribution of this study is that we offer a more fine-tuned explanation for how the diverse construct of chronic pain can impact decision-making, highlighting the aberrant decision-making of an extensive at-risk population. Chronic pain is often a symptom of other chronic conditions, which often require complex management from a diverse team of providers Thus, it is critical for patients to follow their clinicians' recommendations closely; for example, taking their medications as scheduled, complying with nutritional and exercise guidelines, and receiving preventative care for other conditions.

A tendency for immediate gratification over long-term wellbeing is associated with poor health decisions, resulting in obesity, smoking, risky sexual activity, a reduced likelihood for mammography screenings, and a lower probability of adherence with diabetes treatment (9, 12-13). It can be inferred from the results of this study that those with certain types of CP are more likely to engage in these risky behaviors as a result of their PB, which may ultimately compromise their long-term wellbeing. By having a greater awareness of PB, providers may be able to help patients overcome this bias and make decisions that help improve the management of their chronic condition and improve their patients' long-term wellbeing.

Implications

It is beneficial to assess the time preferences of each individual patient with CP, with particular attention to those with high total CP intensity, high intensity continuous CP, or high intensity intermittent CP. If providers can make patients aware of these intrinsic biases, patients can become more aware of them and self-correct their decisions toward choosing options that maximize overall health and long-term wellbeing.

Next, as choice architects, providers can benefit from guiding the conversation about treatment options with patients in a way that best meets their long-term goals. To combat potential time-related biases, the physician can leverage other behavioral economic tools. For example, the physician can utilize anchoring – the tendency for individuals to make decisions revolving around a set starting point (22). Consider the two following encounters:

1. On average a patient with your type and intensity of pain experiments with holistic, non-pharmaceutical therapies before taking opioids.
2. On average a patient with your type and intensity of pain experiments with at *least six weeks* of holistic, non-pharmaceutical therapies before taking opioids.

The addition of the six-week time frame tacitly anchors the patient to trying less risky treatments for at least six weeks. Even if the patient tries the holistic therapy for less than six weeks, they are more likely to persist with this regimen because of their extended expectation.

Limitations and future directions

Our study was subject to several limitations. Although the SurveyMonkey Audience platform has been shown to provide generalizable data, there was no clinical verification that individuals who self-report CP meet the diagnostic criteria for having CP. Thus, the generalizability of the results to medical practice settings may be limited. However, even if a respondent's self-reported CP does not meet the diagnostic criteria for CP (in terms of quality, not duration), it does not necessarily discredit the respondent's self-identification of CP psychogenically. Previous research has shown the subjective interpretation of one's symptomology leads to unique illness behavior, defined as a "dynamic response to changing bodily sensations" (23). Although our study did not utilize a clinically validated CP sample, this sample likely expressed similar preferences and/or behaviors as a clinically-validated sample. Further, the SF-MPQ-2 wording asking individuals to report the CP they have experienced over the past week. It is possible that this instrument did not capture the full host of CP symptoms that an individual experiences across their day-to-day life. A revised wording to account for CP symptoms over the past month may provide more accurate responses. In addition, while the online methods allowed us to survey a demographically representative population, the sample size is not large, limiting the generalizability of the findings.

Finally, in contrast to some behavioral economics studies, the WTA method we used did not involve actual financial incentives, and responses to hypothetical scenarios may not reflect subjects' practical experience.

Future research would benefit from a time preferences instrument that is financially incentivized to more accurately gauge preferences. Moreover, this study focused on the future discounting of positive outcomes (i.e., receiving money). It would be worthwhile to determine whether these results are consistent using scenarios involving discounting of negative future outcomes (i.e., losing money). In addition, including the domain-specificity of other types of stressors and biases (i.e., moral or social stressors) could yield insights into the effects of other vulnerabilities and risks experienced by CP sufferers. Finally, patients whose CP condition has been clinically diagnosed should be studied, to assess the association between their PB and subsequent compliance with clinical treatment recommendations. Such a study would help to validate the link between time preference and health decision making among this population, which will be important to limit dependence on medication therapies for pain.

CONCLUSION

This study asserts that CP impacts decision-making in a variety of type-specific ways. Based on the CP public health crisis and the insufficient understanding of chronic pain patient psychology, results from this study can be used for better treating the hundreds of millions of people suffering CP. By better understanding which types and types-specific intensities of CP are more likely to be associated with PB, clinicians can implement strategies that improve those with CP's choice of and compliance with treatment.

ACKNOWLEDGMENTS

We thank Mandeep Sidhu, MD, James Bennett PhD, Ravneet Bhullar, MD, and Kaywana Raeburn, PhD for their critical feedback and domain-expertise. We thank Amber Stephenson, PhD, and Paul Feustel, PhD, for their assistance in data analysis. The authors have no conflicts of interest to declare. Funding for this project was provided by Albany Medical College. Informed consent was obtained from each individual participant involved in this study. This study was conducted in accordance with the 1964 Declaration of Helsinki and its subsequent amendments.

REFERENCES

[1] Treede R, Rief W, Barke A, Aziz Q, Bennett MI, Benoliel R, et al. Chronic pain as a symptom or a disease. Pain 2019;160(1):19-27. doi:10.1097/j.pain.0000000000001384.

[2] Institute of Medicine of the National Academies. Relieving pain in America: A blueprint for transforming prevention, care, education, and research, 2011. URL: https://www.ncbi.nlm.nih.gov/books/NBK91497/pdf/Bookshelf_NBK91497.pdf.

[3] Davis JA, Robinson RL, Le TK, Xie J. Incidence and impact of pain conditions and comorbid illnesses. J Pain Res 2011;4:331–45. https://doi.org/10.2147/JPR.S24170.

[4] Gaskin DJ, Richard P. The economic costs of pain in the United States. J Pain 2012;13(8):715-24. doi:10.1016/j.jpain.2012.03.009.

[5] van Leeuwen MT, Blyth FM, March LM, Nicholas MK, Cousins MJ. Chronic pain and reduced work effectiveness: The hidden cost to Australian employers. Eur J Pain 2012;10(2):161-6. doi:10.1016/j.ejpain.2005.02.007.

[6] Perlman M, Raeburn K. Investigating the impact of pain type and intensity on risk preferences. Schenectady, NY: Union College, 2019.

[7] Wakaizumi K, Jabakhanji R, Ihara N, Kosugi S, Terasawa Y, Morisaki H, et al. Altered functional connectivity associated with time discounting in chronic pain. Sci Rep 2019;9(1). doi:10.1038/s41598-019-44497-5.

[8] Tompkins DA, Johnson PS, Smith MT, Strain EC, Edwards RR, Johnson MW. Temporal preference in individuals reporting chronic pain: discounting of delayed pain-related and monetary outcomes. Pain 2016;157(8):1724–32. doi.org/10.1097/j.pain.0000000000000576.

[9] Lawless L, Drichoutis AC, Nayga RM. Time preferences and health behaviour: A review. Agric. Food Econ 2013;1(1):1-17. doi:10.1186/2193-7532-1-17.

[10] Green L, Myerson J. A discounting framework for choice with delayed and probabilistic rewards. Psychol Bull 2004;130(5):769-92. doi:10.1037/0033-w2909.130.5.769.

[11] O'donoghue T, Rabin M. Doing it now or later. Am Econ Rev 1999;89(1):103-24. doi:10.1257/aer.89.1.103.

[12] Fang H, Wang Y. Estimating dynamic discrete choice models with hyperbolic discounting, with an application to mammography decisions. Int Econ Rev 2015;56(2):565-96. doi:10.1111/iere.12115.

[13] Wang Y, Sloan FA. Present bias and health. J Risk Uncert 2018;57(2):177–98. doi.org/10.1007/s11166-018-9289-z.

[14] Centers for Disease Control and Prevention. Behavioral risk factor surveillance system. 2018. URL: https://www.cdc.gov/brfss/questionnaires/index.htm.

[15] Dworkin JH, Turk DC, Trudeau JJ, Benson C, Biondi DM, Katz NP, et al. Validation of the revised Short Form McGill Pain Questionnaire (SF-MPQ-2) for self-report of pain qualities in patients with acute low back pain. J Pain Res 2015;13(4):357-66. doi:10.1016/j.jpain.2012.01.022.

[16] Horn C, Blischke Y, Kunz M, Lautenbacher S. Does pain necessarily have an affective component? Negative evidence from blink reflex experiments. Pain Res Manag 2012;17(1):15–24. https://doi.org/10.1155/2012/478019.

[17] Murnion BP. Neuropathic pain: current definition and review of drug treatment. Aust Prescr 2018;41(3):60–3. https://doi.org/10.18773/austprescr.2018.022.

[18] Meier S, Sprenger C. Present-biased preferences and credit card borrowing. Am Econ J Appl Econ 2010;2(1):193–210. doi: 10.1257/app.2.1.193.

[19] Peters E, Slovic P, Gregory R. The role of affect in the WTA/WTP disparity. J Behav Decis Mak 2003;16(4):309-30. doi:10.1002/bdm.448.

[20] Rustøen T, Wahl AK, Hanestad BR, Lerdal A, Paul S, Miaskowski C. Age and the experience of chronic pain: differences in health and quality of life among younger, middle-aged, and older adults. Clin J Pain 2005;21(6):513–23. https://doi.org/10.1097/01.ajp.0000146217.31780.ef.

[21] Colloca L, Ludman T, Bouhassira D, Baron R, Dickenson AH, Yarnitsky D, et al. Neuropathic pain. Nat Rev Dis Primers 2017;3:17002. https://doi.org/10.1038/nrdp.2017.2

[22] Thaler RH, Sunstein CR. Nudge: improving decisions about health, wealth, and happiness. New York: Penguin Books, 2009:1.

[23] Osterweis M, Kleinman A, Mechanic, D. Pain and disability: Clinical, behavioral, and public policy perspectives. Washington, DC: National Academies Press, 1987:146–164.

[24] Coutlee CG, Politzer CS, Hoyle RH, Huettel SA. An Abbreviated Impulsiveness Scale (ABIS) constructed through confirmatory factor analysis of the BIS-11. Arch Scand Psychol 2014;2(1):1–12. doi:10.1037/arc0000005.

[25] Dohmen T, Falk A, Huffman D, Sunde U, Schupp J, Wagner GG. Individual risk attitudes: Measurement, determinants, and behavioral consequences. J Eur Econ Assoc 2011;9(3):522-50. doi:10.1111/j.1542-4774.2011.01015.x.

Appendix: Informed Consent Form

Clarkson University: Documentation of Informed Consent to Participate in Research

Project Title: An Investigation of Preferences about Time

Researcher(s): Marc Perlman and John Huppertz

Institutional Review Board (IRB) approval number: 19-62

Approval valid until: N/A: Continuing Review Waived

You have been asked to be a part of the research described here. Participation is voluntary.

Summary of Study:

We are interested in learning about individuals' attitudes about time in various populations. You will be asked to complete a short survey that will take approximately 12-minutes. There are no foreseeable risks to taking part in this study.

Please read the material below if you are interested in participating in this study.

What to expect:

You will be asked to complete five consecutive surveys asking you to provide demographic information, your current health status, and ways in which you make decisions.

Risks and discomforts to you if you take part in this study:

There are no foreseeable risks or discomforts to you for taking part in this study. However, it is possible that you may experience some minor psychological discomfort in answering some of the questions. If you do, you may skip these questions or you may end the survey without any penalty.

The benefits to you if you take part in this study:

Your responses will be used to improve the medical community by helping to understand implicit biases ingrained in one's health decisions. By better understanding and quantifying these implicit biases, policymakers and physicians can introduce interventions to minimize harmful health decision making.

What will you receive for taking part in this study:

There are no direct benefits of participating in this study.

What will happen to the information collected in this study:

The information collected will be kept confidential as much as is permitted by law. No identifying information will be collected.

What rights you have when you take part in this study:

Participation in this research is voluntary. Deciding not to take part, or to stop being a part of this research will result in no penalty, fine or loss of benefits that you otherwise have a right to. If you have questions about your rights as a research subject or if you wish to report any harm, injury, risk or other concern, please contact the Clarkson University Institutional Review Board (IRB) for human subjects research: (315) 268-6485 or irb@clarkson.edu.

Conflict of Interest: The researchers have no financial interest in performing this study.

Informed Consent: Please check the box below to show you have had the purpose of this research explained and you have been informed of what to expect and your rights. You should have all your questions answered to your satisfaction. Your signature shows that you agree to take part in this research. By signing below, you also attest that you are at least 18 years old. You may take a screen recording of this consent form to keep for your records.

☐

Date ____

Please be aware that you can print or record your screen to save this informed consent form for your records.

A. Survey

Demographic Questionnaire

1) How would you identify your race/ethnicity (check all that apply)?

1. White
2. Black
3. Latino (any race)
4. Asian or Pacific Islander
5. Native American
6. Prefer not to answer
7. Other (Please specify): ______________________

2) What is the highest level of education you have?

1. Did not finish High School
2. High School Diploma or GED
3. Associate's Degree (2-year degree)
4. Vocational Degree
5. Some College
6. Bachelor's Degree (4-year degree)
7. Graduate Degree (Masters, Ph.D, JD, MD, etc)

8. Prefer not to answer
9. Other (Please specify): ______________

3) Would you say that in general your health is—
1) Poor
2) Fair
3) Good
4) Very Good
5) Excellent

4) Do you have chronic pain?
1) Yes
2) No

Short-Form McGill Pain Questionnaire (15)

For this questionnaire, we will provide you a list of words that describe some of the different qualities of pain and related symptoms. Please rate the intensity of each of the pain and related symptoms you felt during the past week on 0 to 10 scale, with 0 being no pain and 10 being the worst pain you can imagine. Use 0 if the word does not describe your pain or related symptoms.

	0	1	2	3	4	5	6	7	8	9	10
Throbbing Pain	○	○	○	○	○	○	○	○	○	○	○
Cramping Pain	○	○	○	○	○	○	○	○	○	○	○
Gnawing Pain	○	○	○	○	○	○	○	○	○	○	○
Aching Pain	○	○	○	○	○	○	○	○	○	○	○
Heavy Pain	○	○	○	○	○	○	○	○	○	○	○
Tender	○	○	○	○	○	○	○	○	○	○	○

	0	1	2	3	4	5	6	7	8	9	10
Shooting Pain	○	○	○	○	○	○	○	○	○	○	○
Stabbing Pain	○	○	○	○	○	○	○	○	○	○	○
Sharp Pain	○	○	○	○	○	○	○	○	○	○	○
Splitting Pain	○	○	○	○	○	○	○	○	○	○	○
Electric-Shock Pain	○	○	○	○	○	○	○	○	○	○	○
Piercing	○	○	○	○	○	○	○	○	○	○	○

	0	1	2	3	4	5	6	7	8	9	10
Tiring-exhausting	○	○	○	○	○	○	○	○	○	○	○
Sickening	○	○	○	○	○	○	○	○	○	○	○
Fearful	○	○	○	○	○	○	○	○	○	○	○
Punishing-cruel	○	○	○	○	○	○	○	○	○	○	○

	0	1	2	3	4	5	6	7	8	9	10
Hot-burning pain	○	○	○	○	○	○	○	○	○	○	○
Cold-freezing pain	○	○	○	○	○	○	○	○	○	○	○
Pain caused by light touch	○	○	○	○	○	○	○	○	○	○	○
Itching	○	○	○	○	○	○	○	○	○	○	○
Tingling or "pins and needles"	○	○	○	○	○	○	○	○	○	○	○
Numbness	○	○	○	○	○	○	○	○	○	○	○

Willingness to Pay Time Preference Survey

Instructions:

The following questions are different from previous ones. All payment amounts are purely hypothetical, however we ask that you make decisions as if you would be getting paid for real.

Decision #1:

Consider the following hypothetical scenario. Imagine you could choose between receiving $500 **right now** OR $X in **1 month**. What is the minimum dollar payment you would be willing to accept to receive that amount in 1 month instead of receiving $500 right now?

$______

Decision #2:

Consider the following hypothetical scenario. Imagine you could choose between receiving $500 **right now** OR $X in **2 months**. What is the minimum dollar payment you would be willing to accept to receive that amount in 2 months instead of receiving $500 right now?

$______

Decision #3:

Consider the following hypothetical scenario. Imagine you could choose between receiving $500 **right now** OR $X in **3 months**. What is the minimum dollar payment you would be willing to accept to receive that amount in 3 months instead of receiving $500 right now?

$______

Decision #4:

Consider the following hypothetical scenario. Imagine you could choose between receiving $500 **in 6 months** OR $X in **7 months**. What is the minimum dollar payment you would be willing to accept to receive that amount in 7 months instead of receiving $500 in 6 months?

$______

Decision #5:

Consider the following hypothetical scenario. Imagine you could choose between receiving $500 **in 6 months** OR $X in **8 months**. What is the minimum dollar payment you would be willing to accept to receive that amount in 8 months instead of receiving $500 in 6 months?

$______

Decision #6:

Consider the following hypothetical scenario. Imagine you could choose between receiving $500 **in 6 months** OR $X in **9 months**. What is the minimum dollar payment you would be willing to accept to receive that amount in 9 months instead of receiving $500 in 6 months?

$______

Abbreviated Impulsiveness Scale (24)

DIRECTIONS: People differ in the ways they act and think in different situations. This is a test to measure some of the ways in which you act and think. Read each statement and put an X on the appropriate circle on the right side of this page. Do not spend too much time on any statement. Answer quickly and honestly.

① Rarely/Never ② Occasionally ③ Often ④ Almost Always/Always

I am a careful thinker.	①	②	③	④
I plan trips well ahead of time.	①	②	③	④
I do things without thinking.	①	②	③	④
I concentrate easily.	①	②	③	④
I plan for job security.	①	②	③	④
I act "on impulse."	①	②	③	④
I am self controlled.	①	②	③	④
I say things without thinking.	①	②	③	④
I don't "pay attention."	①	②	③	④
I act on the spur of the moment.	①	②	③	④
I plan tasks carefully.	①	②	③	④
I am a steady thinker.	①	②	③	④
I am future oriented.	①	②	③	④

Dohmen Single Item Questionnaire (25)

Please answer these questions to the best of your ability. 0 refers to "not at all willing to take risks" and 10 refers to "very willing to take risks."

	0	1	2	3	4	5	6	7	8	9	10
How do you see yourself? Are you **generally** a person who is fully prepared to take risks or do you try to avoid taking risks?	○	○	○	○	○	○	○	○	○	○	○
How would you rate your willingness to take risks **with your health**?	○	○	○	○	○	○	○	○	○	○	○
How would you rate your willingness to take risks **in financial matters**?	○	○	○	○	○	○	○	○	○	○	○

In: Pain Management
Editors: J Merrick and M Morad
ISBN: 978-1-68507-493-7

Chapter 17

FUNCTIONAL RECOVERY PROGRAM AS AN INTERDISCIPLINARY APPROACH TO TREATING CHRONIC PAIN

Kaivalya S Deshpande[1,*], MD, Christian Roehmer[2], MD, George Raum[3], BS and Olga Slavin-Spenny[4], PhD

[1]Department of Physical Medicine and Rehabilitation, University of Pittsburgh Medical Center, Pittsburgh, Pennsylvania, United States of America

[2]Department of Physical Medicine and Rehabilitation, Vanderbilt University Medical Center, Nashville, Tennessee, United States of America

[3]Department of Physical Medicine and Rehabilitation, Philadelphia College of Osteopathic Medicine, Philadelphia, Pennsylvania, United States of America

[4]Ascension Health Michigan Team Rehabilitation, Southfield, Michigan, United States of America

---

* ***Correspondence:*** Kaivalya S Deshpande, MD, University of Pittsburgh Medical Center, Department of Physical Medicine and Rehabilitation, 3471 Fifth Avenue, Suite 910, Pittsburgh, PA 15213, United States. Email: deshpandek@upmc.edu.

ABSTRACT

The Functional recovery program (FRP) models a biopsychosocial approach, utilizing an interdisciplinary team to treat individuals with chronic pain with the aim to improve functioning, develop pain coping strategies, and help patients discontinue pain medications. 53 participants were recruited with chronic low back pain, knee pain, and/or shoulder pain having loss of physical and psychosocial functioning. An evaluation of functional abilities was completed at baseline and at program completion. Mean differences across the assessment metrics were compared using the student's t-test. The chi square test was used to compare participants completing the program with those who chose not to participate on background characteristics. Results: Participants showed significant improvements in functional abilities at program completion and significant decreases in pain-related disability, catastrophizing, pain intensity and interference in activities, and psychological distress (all $p < .01$). Additionally, all participants that completed the program discontinued opioid pain medication. There were no significant differences between those completing the program and those who chose not to participate on any assessed background characteristic. Conclusions: The Functional Recovery Program utilizes a holistic treatment model that provides a structured setting, enabling patients to improve their functioning while better coping with their chronic pain.

INTRODUCTION

Pain affects millions of Americans and continues to contribute to our nation's disability, morbidity, and mortality rates (1). Chronic pain is defined as pain that is persistent or recurrent for a period of 3 months or longer (2). Although statistics vary, it is estimated that 30 to 40 percent of the US adult population are living with chronic pain (3). Chronic pain prevents many individuals from participating in complex activities, reduces their quality of life, and can sometimes cause stigmatization.

When acute pain becomes persistent, it can lead to maladaptive responses and cognitions that may be overlooked in the traditional biomedical models of pain assessments (4). While in the acute stage, pain may be primarily due to tissue damage; as the unresolved issue becomes chronic, physiological changes, such as central sensitization and psychosocial factors (i.e., pain catastrophizing and kinesiophobia), can influence pain perception (5) (see figure 1). One-dimensional treatments targeting only the biomechanical causes of nociception, such as opioids, may not provide effective benefits when a patient's condition becomes chronic (6). Other common therapies for pain include medications such as non-steroidal anti-inflammatories, injections, and surgeries, which are all limited to targeting nociceptive receptors but neglect to address other mechanisms of pain. In the case of opioids, continued reliance on a unimodal approach to treating pain may lead to drug dependence, or even misuse, depending on the progression of the disease and the patient's other psychosocial risk factors (7).

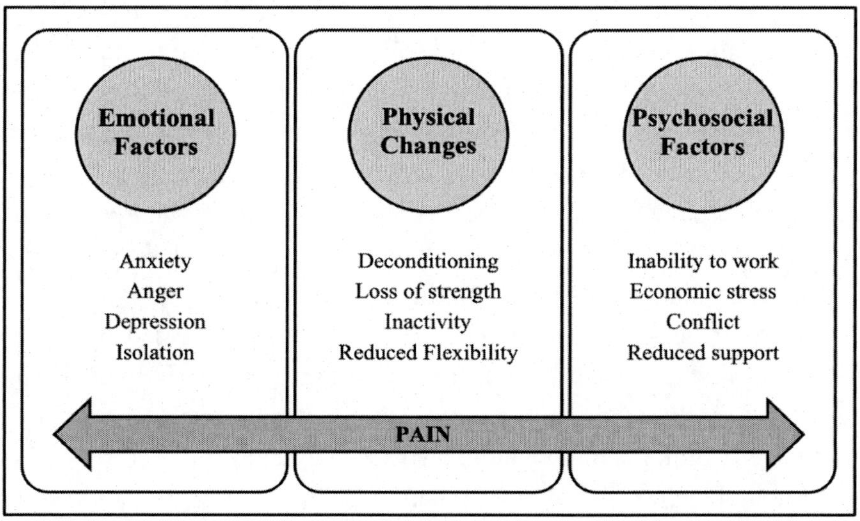

Figure 1. The pain cycle. The pain cycle depicts how psychosocial stressors, emotional factors, and physical changes, feed into each other and contribute to the pain response.

As chronic pain worsens and causes restrictions in patients' ability to work, to socialize, and to care for themselves, it is considered to be "high-impact" chronic pain. "High-impact" pain in patients is associated with increased healthcare expenditures and increased likelihood of opioid abuse

(8). Such pain is associated with more than double the healthcare costs of low-impact chronic pain. Patients with high impact chronic pain are also four times more likely to use opioid medications, and to use them at substantially higher doses than those dealing with low-impact chronic pain (9). Overall, healthcare resource utilization (HRU) and costs involving patients coping with high-impact chronic pain have been shown to increase for the first 6 months after initiating opioid therapies (10).

It is the combination of physical, psychological, and social factors that perpetuates chronic pain. Adapting an interdisciplinary approach which emphasizes all biopsychosocial domains becomes paramount in better understanding and managing chronic pain (11). Traditional multidisciplinary approaches to chronic pain often involve treatments which address specific, separate components and are often implemented without the benefit of having strong communication between care providers. In contrast, an interdisciplinary approach to chronic pain management entails garnering input from various care providers across multiple disciplines who are working cooperatively towards a common goal (12, 13). The interdisciplinary approach is a holistic model within which each provider addresses the biopsychosocial component of pain and provides complementary treatments. Core care teams commonly consist of the patient, physician, psychologist, nurse, physical therapist, and occupational therapist. These teams are often supplemented by experts from other domains such as nutrition, radiology, and social work. Using the interdisciplinary method allows care teams to meet the patients' physical, psychological, social, and vocational needs, as each part of the model complements the other components. This synergistic approach has been deemed to have greater benefits in addressing chronic pain, as opposed to a multidisciplinary approach (14).

The Functional recovery program (FRP) utilizes an interdisciplinary approach in the treatment of chronic pain, with the goal of improving physical and psychological functioning and reducing medication dependence. The functional recovery program designed and utilized in this study consists of four major components: medical management, pain psychology, physical/occupational therapy, and education. The goal of the program was for participants to resume employment, discontinue pain medications, resume recreational/social activities, achieve functional well-being, and manage pain and stress. The objective of this study was to determine the effectiveness of the FRP in accomplishing the aforementioned goals, as well as to investigate the nuances involved in using an interdisciplinary approach to treat chronic pain.

OUR STUDY

53 participants with chronic pain were evaluated for the program under a prospective cohort study design, of which 26 individuals completed the entire program. Participants were recruited from physical medicine and rehabilitation clinics within the state of Michigan with written consent to participate in the program.

The study was run under the guidance and jurisdiction of the Institutional Review Board at Team Rehab. The average age of the subjects was 55 years. Subjects had ongoing low back pain, knee pain, and/or shoulder pain (see Table 1). Inclusion criteria entailed having chronic pain (defined as persistent or recurring pain for three months or greater), and having loss of physical and psychosocial functioning due to pain as evident from medical and psychological intake assessment. Participants who consented to the program attended 4-hour sessions three times a week for a total of seven weeks. Treatment sessions included various components, with a focus on medical management such as tapering opioids, physical and occupational therapy and a guided functional restoration exercise program, psychological counselling addressing trauma and behavioral changes, relaxation and mindfulness exercises, and providing education. Group educational sessions included information on sleep hygiene, body mechanics, drug pathophysiology, goal setting, management of flare-ups, cognitive restructuring, stress management, nutrition, and pain neuroscience education. Goals such as resuming employment and recreational activities, as well as reducing dependence on medications, were set and reinforced during each session.

Table 1. Baseline characteristics of enrolled participants[a]

	Program completers (n = 26)				Program non-completers (n = 27)			
Average Age	55.1				55.8			
Gender	Male	Female			Male	Female		
	9.0	17.0			12.0	15.0		
Ethnicity	Caucasian	African American		Other	Caucasian	African American		Other
	14.0	9.0		3.0	13.0	14.0		0.0
Marital Status	Single	Married		Separated	Single	Married		Separated
	7.0	11.0		8.0	11.0	11.0		5.0
Education	Highschool	College		Post-grad	Highschool	College		Post-grad
	8.0	17.0		1.0	12.0	12.0		2.0
Surgery	Yes	No			Yes	No		
	9.0	13.0			11.0	9.0		
Insurance	Medicare	Medicaid		Other	Medicare	Medicaid		Other
	5.0	3.0		18.0	6.0	7.0		12.0
Work Status	Employed	Not-working		Retired	Employed	Not-working		Retired
	3.0	11.0		12.0	3.0	16.0		8.0
Litigation	Yes	No			Yes	No		
	4.0	20.0			5.0	19.0		
Pain Medication	None	Opioids		Non-opioid	None	Opioids		Non-opioid
	18.0	7.0		2.0	14.0	10.0		3.0
Time since Injury (years)	< 1	1-3	3-6	> 6	< 1	1-3	3-6	> 6
	6.0	8.0	5.0	7.0	6.0	6.0	4.0	6.0

[a]There were no statistically significant differences in any of the measured categories when comparing program completers to program non-completers, $p < 0.5$.

An evaluation of functional abilities and symptom measures was completed at baseline and at program completion. Survey tools were selected based on their validity and accuracy in assessing pain domains (15). Measures included the Patient Health Questionnaire-9 (PHQ9), the General Anxiety Disorder-7 (GAD7), the Oswestry Pain Scale, the Pain Catastrophizing Scale (PCS) and the PEG scale. The PHQ9 was used to gauge the presence and severity of depression. The GAD-7 was used to determine the presence and severity of anxiety. The Oswestry Pain Scale determined each participant's level of pain, and interference with life activities. The Pain Catastrophizing Scale was used to determine the level of exaggerated negative mental state of the participants. The PEG scale is a three-item scale that was used to determine pain severity and interference. Functional or fitness assessments were also taken, looking at the number of pulldowns and squats performed, leg, quadriceps, and biceps lifts with resistance, and endurance on treadmill, track, and dash. Mean differences in metrics across the assessment from baseline to completion were compared using students' t-tests; p<0.05 was considered statistically significant. The chi-squared test was used to compare participants completing the program with those who chose not to participate in relation to their background characteristics. An intention to treat analysis design was also utilized.

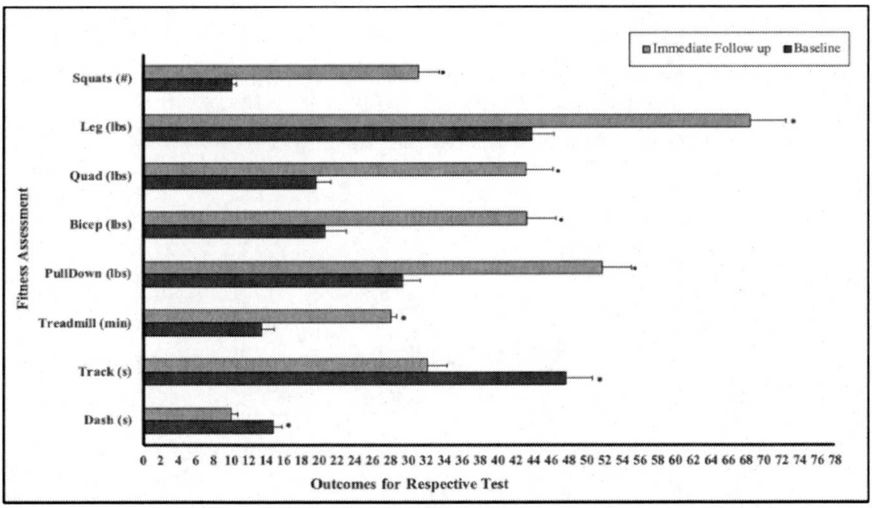

Figure 2. Fitness based assessments. *Indicates statistically significant difference p < 0.5. Assessment metrics amongst various fitness categories tested, including squats, strength testing in legs, quads, biceps and triceps, track, and dash. Measurements taken before and after completion of FRP.

FINDINGS

Participants demonstrated functional improvements across fitness-based assessments in six out of the eight categories tested, including squats, strength testing in legs, quads, biceps and triceps, track, and dash (see Figure 2). Statistically significant improvements were also seen in survey-based assessment scores utilizing the visual analog scale, Generalized Anxiety Scale, Patient Health Questionnaire, Oswestry index, and Pain Catastrophizing Scale upon program completion (see Figure 3). This included decreases in pain-related disability, catastrophizing, pain intensity and interference in activities, and psychological distress.

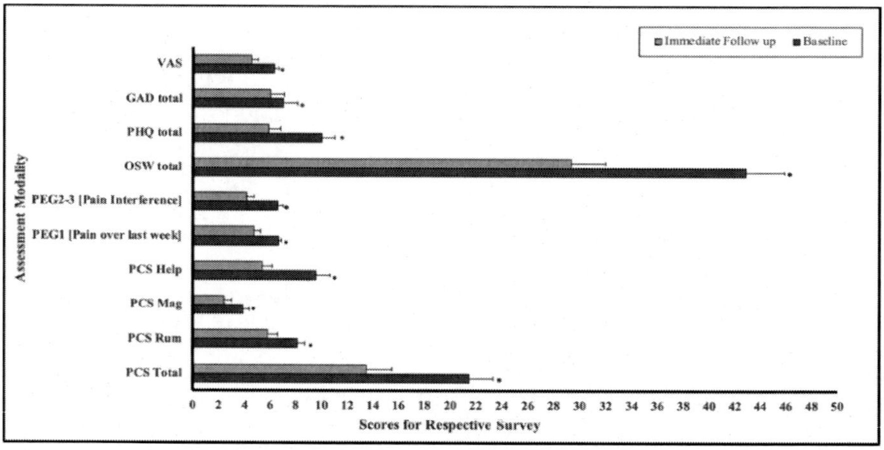

Figure 3. Survey based assessments. *Indicates statistically significant difference p < 0.5. VAS: Visual Analogue Scale; GAD: Generalized Anxiety Disorder Scale; PHQ: Patient Health Questionnaire Scale; OSW: Oswestry Scale; PCS Help: Pain Catastrophizing Scale (Helplessness); PCS Mag: Pain Catastrophizing Scale (Magnification); PCS: Rum: Pain Catastrophizing Scale (Rumination); PCS Total: Pain Catastrophizing Scale Total. Self-reported survey metrics measured before and after completion of FRP, assessing various validated pain, depression, and anxiety domains.

Specific baseline characteristics assessed included demographics, age, injury location, previous surgery, socioeconomic status, and insurance. There were no significant differences between those completing the program and those who failed to complete the program on any assessed background characteristics (see Table 1. Nine of the patients that completed the program were on maintenance doses of opioid medications ranging from 2.5 to 40 morphine equivalents per day and were all weaned off of the medications by program completion.

DISCUSSION

The functional recovery program (FRP) was developed as an interdisciplinary, multimodal treatment approach for patients with chronic pain. The program goals included the following: that patients resume employment, discontinue pain medications, resume recreational/social activities, achieve functional well-being, and appropriately manage pain and stress. The study demonstrates that the FRP was largely able to help patients achieve these goals.

Interdisciplinary programs, such as the FRP, utilize patient-centered biopsychosocial treatment strategies which incorporate health education, physical, vocational, and psychological components, targeting all proposed mechanisms of the chronic pain process. Interdisciplinary programs have drawn researchers' interest due to increased acceptance of the biopsychosocial model of pain, as well as the inadequacies of monotherapy in relieving pain. Indeed, interdisciplinary models have been found to be more effective than multidisciplinary approaches, which effectuate treatments in a siloed, disconnected manner (16). Recent studies reflect that interdisciplinary models result in better outcomes for lower back pain, emotional and physical function, and work capacity (17, 18). As one of the few interdisciplinary treatment programs in the country, FRP was built to expand upon prior studies; it emphasizes the importance of functional restoration and cognitive behavioral pain management, with a focus on resolving the negative consequences of pain and changing the behavior and reaction patterns secondary to treatment refractory pain.

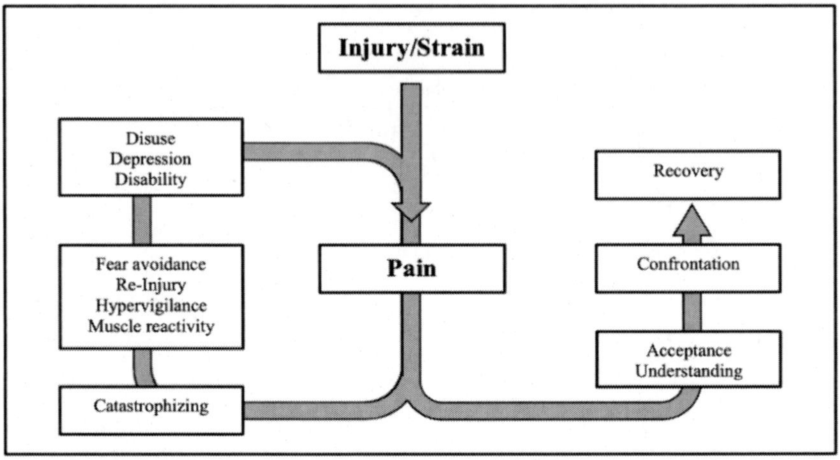

Figure 4. The pain behavioral arc. The pain behavioral arc illustrates the self-perpetuating nature of chronic pain and how maladaptive behaviors can lead to persistence of the pain response. In contrast, early confrontation and corrective adaptations can allow for detachment from the arc and promote recovery.

In an effort to break detrimental pain behavior arcs (see Figure 4), a main priority during FRP sessions was placed on neuroscience pain education. The education was meant to help patients better manage their pain, mitigating catastrophizing and kinesiophobia. Many past educational models for pain have focused on the anatomical and biomechanical models for explaining the source of pain to a patient. However, studies have shown that these older models may not be the most effective way to direct pain education and may even lead to patients having increased stress and anxiety related to their pain (19). In contrast, neuroscience pain education models have shown to be effective in mitigating avoidance behaviors (20, 21). The educational emphasis in FRP was placed on highlighting differences in pain caused by tissue damage versus centralized pain, which helped patients understand that they would not be at risk by doing physical exercises and completing ADLs. The neuroscience pain education emphasis also enabled patients to normalize their feelings of discomfort while completing various tasks. In addition, the model used in FRP focused on reviewing patient imaging and addressing misconceptions that patients had regarding their conditions, while avoiding the use of degenerative terms in patient discussions. Patients' negative perceptions about their bodies further contribute to the neuropsychological phenomena leading to their pain, possibly resulting in further disability and chronicity (22).

Decreased pain avoidance behaviors and increased activity levels resulted when caregivers helped patients understand their symptoms during therapy. Significant improvements in patients' scores on the Visual Analogue Scale, Generalized Anxiety Disorder Scale, Patient Health Questionnaire, and Pain Catastrophizing Scales were noted upon completion of the program. Likely secondary to these findings, participants were able to successfully complete their physical and occupational therapy sessions, showing improvements in an average of 6 out of 8 fitness assessments. Overall, these physical gains translated into improvements in self-reported functional abilities, with a significant decrease in the Oswestry Scale, a validated scale for scoring LBP and resulting disability.

Another major benefit of the FRP program was participants' decreased reliance on pharmacotherapy, specifically opiates. As the opioid crisis continues to be a major problem in the United States, the use of non-opiate modalities must continue to be encouraged. The National Survey on Drug Use and Health in 2015 revealed that approximately 36% of adults in the U.S. admitted to having taken an opioid within the prior year, and that 13% of that sample admitted to not having used the drug as prescribed. As of 2017, there were 33,000 deaths per year due to misuse of prescription and illegal opioids (23). FRP proved to be effective toward patients' complete discontinuation of opiates after seven weeks, indicating that the program may be useful as a modality to limit patients' opiate use.

LIMITATIONS

There are several limitations in this study that merit discussion. While functional rehabilitation programs for pain target many aspects of the biopsychosocial model effectively, there are some characteristics of these programs that hinder widespread use. Within this study of 53 participants, 27 were lost to follow-up or dropped out of the program prior to completion. Interestingly, external factors such as demographics, socioeconomic status, employment, injury, and medications being used by participants did not play a statistically significant role in the dropout rate. It should be noted that the program has a high resource burden that requires dedicated compliance and commitment from participants. Future research could help in predicting the likelihood of participation, as well as improving methods for engaging patients in interdisciplinary rehabilitation programs. An additional limitation in this study was that it did not stratify patients by type of pain. Although the program was statistically significant overall for treating pain, future studies should look to delineate participants by pain etiologies to determine the pathologies for which FRP may be most effective. Furthermore, although all the objective survey scores in this study were statistically significant, their clinical significance may vary, and this was not assessed. The use of an appropriately matched randomized control comparing patients that did not undergo the FRP should also be utilized to better demonstrate the validity of using such an approach to treat chronic pain.

Lastly, a historical deterrent of interdisciplinary models, are the up-front costs associated with these approaches. Importantly, several recent studies indicate that while the cost of utilizing an interdisciplinary approach for chronic pain may exceed traditional therapies in the short-term, over the course of treatment, total costs may be reduced due to the resulting decreased need for more invasive options (24, 25). Of note, many of the patients enrolled in this study were nearing the point where they were set to undergo additional invasive treatments, such as injections and/or surgeries. Further studies should investigate the cost-effectiveness of an interdisciplinary program versus more invasive options.

Conclusion

Chronic/centralized pain is a complex problem that often warrants a different treatment approach than acute/peripheral pain. The functional recovery program provides a structured setting that enables patients to improve pain control, reduce medication compliance, and attain improvement of function. External factors such as demographics, socioeconomic status, employment, injury, and medications used by participants did not have a statistically significant influence on the dropout rate. By utilizing the biopsychosocial treatment model, providers can expand upon current strategies, helping patients with chronic pain to achieve a better quality of life.

ACKNOWLEDGMENTS

Disclosure/conflict of interest: The authors whose names are listed above certify that they have NO conflict or affiliations with or involvement in any organization or entity with any financial interest (such as honoraria; educational grants; participation in speakers' bureaus; membership, employment, consultancies, stock ownership, or other equity interest; and expert testimony or patent-licensing arrangements), or non-financial interest (such as personal or professional relationships, affiliations, knowledge or beliefs) in the subject matter or materials discussed in this manuscript.

This manuscript has not been published elsewhere and is not under consideration by any other journals. Data from this manuscript was accepted as part of an abstract and was presented in the form of an oral presentation at the 2019 American Academy of Pain Medicine conference in Colorado.

Funding: No funding sources were received for this study. This study was conducted in accordance with the 1964 Declaration of Helsinki and its subsequent amendments. Informed consent was obtained from each individual participant involved in this study.

REFERENCES

[1] Mokdad AH, Ballestros K, Echko M, Glenn S, Olsen HE, Mullany E, et al. The state of US health, 1990-2016. JAMA 2018;319:1444.

[2] Treede R-D, Rief W, Barke A, Aziz Q, Bennett MI, Benoliel R, et al. A classification of chronic pain for ICD-11. Pain 2015;1.

[3] Dahlhamer J, Lucas J, Zelaya , Carla, Nahin R, Mackey S, DeBar L, et al. Prevalence of chronic pain and high-impact chronic pain among adults — united states, 2016. MMWR 2018;67:1001–6.

[4] Dansie EJ, Turk DC. Assessment of patients with chronic pain. Br J Anaesth 2013;111:19–25.

[5] Niederstrasser NG, Meulders A, Meulders M, Slepian PM, Vlaeyen JWS, Sullivan MJL. Pain catastrophizing and fear of pain predict the experience of pain in body parts not targeted by a delayed-onset muscle soreness procedure. J Pain 2015;16:1065–76.

[6] Chaparro LE, Furlan AD, Deshpande A, Mailis-Gagnon A, Atlas S, Turk DC. opioids compared with placebo or other treatments for chronic low back pain. Spine 2014;39:556–63.

[7] Pergolizzi J, Ahlbeck K, Aldington D, Alon E, Coluzzi F, Dahan A, et al. The development of chronic pain: physiological change necessitates a multidisciplinary approach to treatment. Curr Med Res Opin 2013;29:1127–35.

[8] Herman PM, Edgington SE, Ryan GW, Coulter ID. Prevalence and characteristics of chronic spinal pain patients with different hopes (treatment goals) for ongoing chiropractic care. J Altern Complement Med 2019;25:1015–25.

[9] Herman PM, Broten N, Lavelle TA, Sorbero ME, Coulter ID. Health care costs and opioid use associated with high-impact chronic spinal pain in the United States. Spine 2019;44:1154–61.

[10] Kern D, Zhou S, Chavoshi S, Tunceli O, Sostek M, Singer J, et al. Treatment patterns, healthcare utilization, and costs of chronic opioid treatment for non-cancer pain in the united states. Am J Manag Care 2015;21:222–34.

[11] Farre A, Rapley T. The new old (and old new) medical model: four decades navigating the biomedical and psychosocial understandings of health and illness. Healthcare 2017;5:88.

[12] Martín J, Torre F, Padierna A, Aguirre U, González N, García S, et al. six-and 12-month follow-up of an interdisciplinary fibromyalgia treatment programme: results of a randomised trial. Clin Exp Rheumatol 2012;30:103–11.

[13] Quintner JL, Cohen ML, Buchanan D, Katz JD, Williamson OD. Pain medicine and its models: helping or hindering? Pain Med 2008;9:824–34.

[14] Scascighini L, Toma V, Dober-Spielmann S, Sprott H. Multidisciplinary treatment for chronic pain: a systematic review of interventions and outcomes. Rheumatology 2008;47:670–8.

[15] Krebs EE, Lorenz KA, Bair MJ, Damush TM, Wu J, Sutherland JM, et al. Development and initial validation of the peg, a three-item scale assessing pain intensity and interference. J Gen Intern Med 2009;24:733–8.

[16] Collins FS, Koroshetz WJ, Volkow ND. Helping to end addiction over the long-term. JAMA 2018;320:129.

[17] Takahashi N, Kasahara S, Yabuki S. Development and implementation of an inpatient multidisciplinary pain management program for patients with intractable chronic musculoskeletal pain in Japan: preliminary report. J Pain Res 2018;11:201–11.

[18] Takahashi N, Takatsuki K, Kasahara S, Yabuki S. Multidisciplinary pain management program for patients with chronic musculoskeletal pain in Japan: a cohort study. J Pain Res 2019;12:2563–76.

[19] Schultz R, Smith J, Newby JM, Gardner T, Shiner CT, Andrews G, et al. Pilot trial of the reboot online program: an internet-delivered, multidisciplinary pain management program for chronic pain. Pain Res Manag 2018;2018:1–11.

[20] Louw A, Diener I, Butler DS, Puentedura EJ. The effect of neuroscience education on pain, disability, anxiety, and stress in chronic musculoskeletal pain. Arch Phys Med Rehabil 2011;92:2041–56.

[21] Louw A, Nijs J, Puentedura EJ. A clinical perspective on a pain neuroscience education approach to manual therapy. J Man Manip Ther 2017;25:160–8.

[22] Sloan TJ, Walsh DA. Explanatory and diagnostic labels and perceived prognosis in chronic low back pain. Spine 2010;35:E1120–5.

[23] Soelberg CD, Brown RE, du Vivier D, Meyer JE, Ramachandran BK. The US opioid crisis. Anesth Analg 2017;125:1675–81.

[24] Jonas WB, Crawford C, Colloca L, Kriston L, Linde K, Moseley B, et al. Are invasive procedures effective for chronic pain? A systematic review. Pain Med 2019;20:1281–93.

[25] Mahrer NE, Gold JI, Luu M, Herman PM. A cost-analysis of an interdisciplinary pediatric chronic pain clinic. J Pain 2018;19:158–65.

SECTION THREE: CASE STUDIES

In: Pain Management
Editors: J Merrick and M Morad
ISBN: 978-1-68507-493-7

Chapter 18

MIGRAINE WITH EYE PAIN: A CASE OF ALLODYNIA AND EXPERIENTIAL AVOIDANCE

J Carmelo Visdómine-Lozano*[*], *PhD
Instituciones Penitenciarias, Madrid, Spain

ABSTRACT

Migraine is one of the most prevalent disorders related with chronic pain. This paper describes a case of an atypical migraine beginning with pain on the left eye. The objective of this case report is to analyze in a clinical setting the evolution, management and change of an idiosyncratic migraine and the hyperalgesia and allodynia processes involved. One 41 years old patient served to collect relevant data through narrative self-registers during a period of two years. Results show how pain could have its origin in an episode of infection by the virus influenza type A, but later appeared in the form of migraine on conditions of menace and fear of visual damage produced by LEDs. In addition, migraines drastically transformed into diffuse and low-frequency headaches after the change of the psychological function of LEDs as menace. We conclude that

[*] Corresponding Author's Emails: JCarmelo.Visdomine@dgip.mir.es; jcvisdo@gmail.com.

migraines can be the product of hyper-defensive responses of both the central and peripheral nervous systems (hyperalgesia and allodynia), potentiated and expanded by psychological avoidance, beliefs of damage, and even inappropriate pharmacological treatments.

INTRODUCTION

The migraine of the case reported herein appeared without auras, but beginning with pain on the left eye, and thus it can serve as approach to an idiosyncratic type of migraine. Pain is defined as "an unpleasant sensation resulting from the intricate interplay between sensory and cognitive mechanisms" that serves an organism to avoid direct external injuries or to signal inner organs dysfunctions in some cases. Consequently, pain can be classified as nociceptive or neuropathic, depending on the origin of the painful stimulation. Nociceptive pain derives from the activation of peripheral receptors by noxious stimuli, and neuropathic pain is activated as an inflammatory-like response as result of previous illnesses or as consequence of some undetermined circumstance (1). Therefore, neuropathic pain embraces a wide range of pain-related conditions that must be carefully diagnosed. When the pathways of pain transmission generate a sustained sensitization then we talk of chronic pain.

Specifically, migraine is a chronic pain defined as a painful syndrome or idiopathic headache of unknown aetiology, or, at least, of multiple pathogenic origin. Accordingly, migraine could be included in the category of neuropathic pain. Some studies have proposed that this kind of neuropathic pain can be produced by the consumption of substances like caffeine, cheese, alcohol, or chocolate; however, other studies have even centred on arterial hypertension as a risk factor. There does not exist consensus about it (2). Thus, meanwhile some authors think that some oxidative proteins are the responsible for activating migraines, other authors consider that unbalances of some sort of amines are the responsible (2).

So, though the molecular mechanisms of pain are well known nowadays, the triggering factors are not, mainly in neuropathic pain. But, curiously, just from such molecular mechanisms of pain transmission we can excerpt some fundamental conclusions. It is widely accepted that repeated or prolonged direct noxious stimuli provoke both peripheral and central sensitizations through a chained process of enhanced depolarization of nociceptors sodium channels, intracellular increase of calcium levels produced by NMDA and neuropeptide receptors, as well as gene expression promoting long-term shifts in the activation threshold of the nociceptors. In neuropathic pain, immune cells react to the activation of nerve fibres and unchain active microglia of the spinal cord, which, through neurotrophic factors such as GABA and glycine, provoke reductions of inhibitory interneurons, and change the general central modulation of pain transmission. In sum, both processes, and this is the key, are unfolded as sensitization mechanisms which produce "hyperalgesia", that is, a decrease in the threshold of pain activation; and "allodynia", or a generalized "painful" response to non-noxious stimuli" (3).

Hyperalgesia and allodynia are, therefore, crucial processes that allow us to understand pain as a holistic response of an organism, response that functions as a defensive and general anticipation, but that when it is generalized to some extent, then it can involve a serious invalidating situation. Indeed, to have a more complete account of pain, hyperalgesia and allodynia must be considered "learning processes" of the organism. Thus, a complementary perspective must be employed to study such pain mechanisms, for when both hyperalgesia and allodynia mechanisms are not suitably understood, professionals, to our view, can fail in the identification of the origin, evolution, and resistance to pharmacological interventions of pain and migraines in a large amount of cases.

Such complementary perspective is not new or improvised, and leans on several studies concerned on the learned nature of some fundamental variables related with pain (4). Such studies show how both classical and operant conditioning are involved in nocebo effects and hyperalgesia. At this regard, a clinical diagnosis derived from the research on classical and operant learning processes that result in misadjusted behaviours and troublesome experiences, labelled "experiential avoidance", must be conceived a key element among such fundamental variables, as we will try to show with the case reported in this article. Briefly, experiential avoidance can be defined as a verbally-regulated behavioural process by which an individual seeks to eliminate uncomfortable experiences, but that, contrary to the individual's attempts, it basically works potentiating and extending such aversive experiences as a consequence of negative reinforcement. It has even been demonstrated that when this potentiation by experiential avoidance happens with painful stimuli, then pain sensitization appears (5), confirming the relation between avoidance and chronic pain.

In the following sections we will examine the course and evolution of a single clinical case that can help to clarify this situation in a patient diagnosed of an atypical migraine with pain on the left eye, but without auras. Data were collected through narrative self-registers during a period of two years, and the aim of this case report is to show how allodynia and hyperalgesia mechanisms of pain amplification are a consequence of the strengthening and generalization mechanisms of experiential avoidance, rejecting reductionist views of migraines.

CASE REPORT

Chief complaint. The patient (C) was a 41 years old male who reported migraines and headaches beginning with pain on the left eye, but without auras and scintillating scotomas, contrary to usual patients' complaints. His migraines evolved until provoking nausea and vomiting.

C weighed 125 pounds (57 kg) and was 5.6 feet (172 cm) tall. He was married and had three sons. He was diagnosed of hypermetropy (0.25 dioptries on the right eye and 0.75 on the left eye) when he was eleven, after one of his teachers realised that C. turn cross-eyed when looked at the blackboard. Conversely, when he was thirty, he was diagnosed of myopia (0.75 dioptries on both eyes). He was diagnosed of extra-systolic arrhythmias when he was thirty nine, but he was not subjected to pharmacological treatments at the moment in which the migraines appeared. His blood pressure was of 120/81 mmHg, and the patient had neither familial antecedents of neurological disorders, nor other personal relevant medical conditions regarded with eyes or brain illnesses, although he had suffered an infection of the virus Influenza type A four years earlier to the appearance of the migraines, which coursed occasionally with acute pain in the left eye during episodes of high fever. Despite this event did not repeat along the following four years after the infection recovery, it could contribute to explain the allodynia mechanisms underlying the case, as we will see.

C suffered sporadic parietal and occipital headaches along his adolescence, which he attributed to the fact of rejecting the use of glasses. However, he started to suffer serious episodes of migraine that always began with pain on the left eye, when his workplace changed the lighting system, and substituted fluorescents for LEDs. He was 40 years old in that moment, and from then on, he was developing thoughts about the damages produced on the eyes by LED-based technologies (e.g., new workplace lights, new PC monitor, smart phones, new streetlights, etc.), and he attempted to avoid excessive exposure to such lighting sources. C searched information and multiple studies about the damages of LEDs on the retinal cells, and sent an inform to the department of occupational risks; he bought and installed a yellow filter on his PC screen, and when he noted some bothersome sensation on eyes, he closed them and made ocular movements in an attempt to avoid upcoming pain sensations. Finally, he turn to use his glasses after ten years, but migraines grew and eye pain were more frequent than ever, to the extent that he suffered some episodes of nauseas and vomiting that made him going to bed, with the maximum frequency of twice in a month. In two occasions he took aspirin, although as migraines with ocular pain went on, he opted for going to visit an ophthalmologist.

Physical examination results. C went first to an ophthalmologist who examined pupil response, blood vessels of the retina and optic nerve; eyelid, cornea and conjunctiva, as well as eye pressure by a usual tonometry procedure. The results were that C did not suffer any ophthalmologic problem. However, migraines with pain on the eyes continued, and C visited a second ophthalmologist after his first episode of eye pain and vomiting, and the result of this examination was identical to the first ophthalmologic exam. Notwithstanding, he was diagnosed of "dry eye" and "migraine", and this time the ophthalmologist prescribed sodium hyaluronate (SH). C employed SH once or twice per week at the beginning, but since eye pain and subsequent migraines were increasing after any use of his phone, working with his PC, watching TV, or even after a long distance travel on car, he also increased his use of SH up to a frequency of once or twice per day. Three weeks later C suffered migraines of nocturnal occurrence accompanied of pain on the external ear. After two new episodes of nausea and vomiting, C went to a general physician, who prescribed blood and hormonal analysis, although the results did not show anything abnormal. Only bilirubin level was somewhat high (1.1 mg/dL) but inside the range of normality. This doctor diagnosed "migraine", prescribed dexketoprofen, and refused to derive C. to a neurologist due to the low frequency of vomiting, in his opinion, and conversely, decided to derive C to a new ophthalmologist, who also diagnosed "dry eye" and recommended him to continue the use of SH.

Treatment and actual outcome. The treatment in this case can be conceptualized as an example of "bibliotherapy". The patient read a book written by a neurologist who proposed a different perspective about migraines, and C reported a change of perspective towards his pain. This perspective consisted of considering pain as an "alarm system" of the brain that is activated by circumstances with menace functions, but that do not necessarily involve damage. From that moment on, the frequency and intensity of migraines changed drastically. Only in one episode after the reading of this book, C suffered migraine with nausea and vomiting (one week later, approximately). Headaches decreased in intensity, the time interval between pain episodes increased, and the conditions related to them changed from the use of LED-based technologies to different types of stress situations.

Conclusion and Discussion

In the case presented we can see that the course of pain and migraines did not change after pharmacological interventions in the form of analgesics or eye drops; quite the contrary, these interventions increased pain episodes up to nausea, vomiting, and going to bed. Instead, migraines originally triggered by pain on the left eye transformed towards diffuse headaches with decreased intensity after a change of the psychological function of LEDs for the patient. Such function changed from menacing to irrelevant after C read a neurologist's book. The patient learned to consider his pain as a conditioned "alarm system", and from that moment on, he ceased his attempts of avoiding LED-based lighting systems, and other related conditions, such as the belief of that excessive ocular work leads to "dry eye", and "dry eye" to "eye pain". Eyes have their own automatic protective mechanisms which fundamentally are tears. When some noxious or irritant agent is in contact with the eye surface, lacrimal glands secrete tears, and only some specific pathological conditions produce less lacrimal fluid, and then "dry eye" or "keratoconjunctivitis sicca". Such pathological conditions are, for example, "dacryoadenitis" and "Sjögren's syndrome" (6), however, they are accompanied by other symptoms not present in the case described; in fact, they were not diagnosed to C. Consequently, we think that a generic diagnosis of "dry eye" should be avoided in clinical practice, since it is a condition related to more complex and specific ophthalmologic anomalies.

Still, a condition that could help to explain the genesis of pain was the infection of the virus Influenza type A suffered by C four years earlier to the migraines. During this infection, C had acute eye pain, and this could serve as an aversive unconditioned stimulus for the conditioning of some menacing situations for the patient. Whether we take into account that C developed beliefs of menace about eyes damages related to some lighting situations, it is a feasible hypothesis that such beliefs, to the extent that beliefs in this context can be conceived as verbal stimuli (5), activated eye pain as an alarm directed to avoid such (unreal) damages. Hyperalgesia and allodynia, developed once such conditioning took place, facilitated and extended the appearance of pain, while the experiential avoidance of lights and situations of ocular work served to make chronic his eye pain and migraines.

Thus, according to the case reported we propose that pain is a biological response that can be triggered by a wide range of conditions, and that is a process susceptible of participating in classical and operant conditioning due to its very nature and features. Hyperalgesia and allodynia are essential features of pain itself, and both prepare the organism to rapidly response in novel and menacing situations through conditioning processes. We think that views of migraines as products of some type of substances like foods and drinks, or as a consequence of genetic unbalances of amines in the Central Nervous System, are reductionist and do not reflect a proper analysis of the physiological and neurocognitive mechanisms of pain. Perhaps, the cultural belief that establishes that such foods and drinks (as well as other stimuli) are a menace of damage for the organism, is the greatest "painful-genic" factor, at least in cases similar to that reported in this article.

Acknowledgements

This study has not been funded by any public or private institution. The author declare no conflict of interest. Informed consent was obtained and this study was conducted in accordance with the 1964 Declaration of Helsinki and its subsequent amendments.

References

[1] Mumenthaler M, Mattler H, Taub E. Fundamentals of neurology. An illustrated guide. New York: Thieme, 2006.

[2] Lee MJ, Park B, Cho S, Park H, Kim S, Chung C. Dynamic functional connectivity of the migraine brain: a resting-state functional magnetic resonance imaging study. Pain 2019;160(12):2776-86.

[3] Jensen TS, Finnerup NB. Allodynia and hyperalgesia in neuropathic pain: clinical manifestations and mechanisms. Lancet Neurol 2014;13(9):924-35.
[4] Bräscher A, Witthöft M, Becker S. The underestimated significance of conditioning in placebo hypoalgesia and nocebo hyperalgesia. Pain Res Manag 2018;2018:6841985. doi.org/10.1155/ 2018/6841985.
[5] Gutierrez O, Luciano C, Rodriguez M, Fink BC. Comparison between an acceptance-based and a cognitive-control-based protocol for coping with pain. Behav Ther 2004;35(4):767-84.
[6] Khurana A. Comprehensive ophthalmology. New Delhi: New Age Publishers, 2007.

In: Pain Management
Editors: J Merrick and M Morad
ISBN: 978-1-68507-493-7

Chapter 19

ATYPICAL HEMANGIOMAS RESEMBLING METASTASES

Victoria Rico[1], BSc(C), Marjorie Monteiro Rodrigues[1], MD, Dominic Chan[1], MBBS, Yasmeen Razvi[1], BSc(C), Erin McKenzie[1], BSc(C), Henry Lam[1], MRT, Carlo De Angelis[1], PharmD, Edward Chow[1], MBBS and Fiona Lim[2,*], MBBS

[1]Sunnybrook Odette Cancer Centre, University of Toronto, Toronto, Ontario, Canada

[2]Princess Margaret Hospital, Hong Kong, PR China

ABSTRACT

Hemangiomas of the bone account for 1% of all tumors found in the bone. Often asymptomatic in nature, many bone hemangiomas go undetected; however, when they are found on imaging, atypical-looking hemangiomas may be misdiagnosed as metastases in radiology. Methods: The present manuscript reports the case of a 50-year-old

* Corresponding Author's Email: fionalimmy@gmail.com.

woman with a history of breast cancer presenting with a lesion at the T7 vertebra that was initially suspicious for a metastasis, but was later confirmed to be a vertebral bone hemangioma. A literature search with key words 'hemangioma' and 'metastases' was conducted on October 26, 2018 on Ovid Medline (1946 to October Week 2 2018) and Embase (1947 to 2018 week 43) to identify cases where bone hemangiomas were initially mistaken for bone metastases due to close resemblance. Results: Eighteen cases identified from the literature met the inclusion criteria for this review, in addition to the case from our centre as described above. The average age of patients included in this review was 56.7 years. Nine of 19 cases (47.4%) were prior to the diagnosis of bone hemangioma, while the remainder of the cases (n=10, 52.6%) reported symptoms which led to medical imaging and tests, and a final diagnosis of bone hemangioma. Relevant scans and tests, as well as follow-up information are described in detail. Conclusion: Determining optimal diagnostic methods and treatment protocols for bone hemangiomas should be a target for future investigation.

INTRODUCTION

Hemangiomas are benign vascular neoplasms composed of newly formed vessels or proliferated vessel walls and can occur anywhere in the human body(1). Bone hemangiomas represent 1% of all tumors found in the bone, and most commonly occur in the vertebrae and skull (2). There are four histological types of bone hemangiomas which include cavernous, capillary, arteriovenous, and venous (3). Hemangiomas arising in the bone are considered rare, however it is likely that many go undetected because of their slow growing and asymptomatic nature. Often, they are incidentally detected during radiographic examination of other lesions (1). In other cases, bone hemangiomas may produce symptoms, such as pain, visible or palpable alterations to the lesioned bone, and less commonly, osteomalacia, defined as delayed or defective mineralization of the bone, with bone fractures (4, 5) or spinal compression which may subsequently lead to neurological complications and deficits (6).

Undergoing staging evaluation is an essential step following a cancer diagnosis, as detecting or ruling out metastases based on these evaluations guides treatment plans and defines the intent of treatment for patients (7).

In some cases however, benign entities, such as hemangiomas, may resemble metastases, potentially leading to unnecessary treatments including radiation therapy or chemotherapy (8).

Hemangiomas can usually be identified by their distinct appearance on radiography. Generally, hemangiomas have parallel line densities on x-ray due to their thickened vertical trabeculae (9, 10). Typical vertebral hemangioma appearances may be described as "corduroy cloth" due to the vertical striations, while a striated "honeycomb" or "sunburst" pattern is typical for hemangiomas of the skull (11). However, making a definitive diagnosis for bone hemangiomas can be difficult when they appear as atypical. Features found on magnetic resonance imaging (MRI) are largely impacted by the amount of vascularity and fat that compose the lesions. Areas of high signal intensity in T1-weighted MRI are due to high-fat content, and areas of high signal intensity in T2-weighted MRI are due to vascularity of lesions (12). Typical hemangiomas show high-intensity on T1 and T2-weighted images on MRI, as well as coarsened vertical trabeculae on computed tomography (CT) and radiographic imaging(13). On axial CT scans, hemangiomas of the spine would appear as having a "polka dot" pattern (14). Further, CT scans of hemangiomas in the metaphysis and epiphysis of the long bones typically appear as lytic lesions with spiculated pattern (14). Atypical hemangiomas appear hypointense on T1-weighted MRI but have the typical characteristics usually seen in T2-weighted images (15). This atypical appearance may look like a metastatic lesion which usually has low T1-weighted signals, while having high T2-weighted signals on MRI (16). On bone scintigraphy, bone hemangiomas may appear as photopenic and they may also have a moderate increase in radiotracer uptake (17).

The present manuscript describes a patient treated at our centre for breast cancer with an identified lesion at T7 that was suspicious for a metastasis. Upon further investigation the lesion was favoured to be a bone hemangioma. All available literature on bone hemangiomas resembling metastases or being misdiagnosed as metastases are systematically reviewed below (3, 10, 22–27, 11, 14, 15, 17–21). To our knowledge, this is the first literature review of its kind. This review aims to examine commonalities between these atypical hemangiomas, as well as imaging techniques that may be used to aid in a more accurate diagnosis of hemangiomas.

CASE REPORT

A 50-year-old perimenopausal woman presented with self-detected right breast mass with occasional pain and burning sensation at the site of the mass. A right breast ultrasound revealed an irregular solid 2.6 cm mass, suspicious for malignancy, with a Breast Imaging Reporting and Data System (BI-RADS) score of 4. She then had a bilateral mammogram which revealed a 3.2 cm mass in the upper-outer right breast at the site of the questioned palpable lump. A second bilateral mammogram revealed a 3.3 cm spiculated mass in the upper outer right breast with prominent lymph nodes anterior to the mass. A 0.5 cm obscured mass medial to the dominant mass was also observed.

The patient underwent an ultrasound guided biopsy of the index lesion, and pathological analysis revealed a well-differentiated invasive ductal carcinoma with no lymphovascular invasion (LVI). The biomarkers were estrogen receptor (ER) and progesterone receptor (PR) positive, and human epidermal growth factor receptor 2 (HER2) negative.

She underwent a right-sided, skin-sparing, simple mastectomy with sentinel lymph node biopsy (SLNB) and immediate reconstruction with a deep inferior epigastric perforators flap. The mastectomy specimen revealed 11 foci of multifocal invasive ductal carcinoma, with the largest foci being 3.5 cm. The specimen was of low grade with a minor DCIS component. The margins of the invasive carcinoma and the DCIS were clear. Two intramammary lymph nodes were positive with macrometastasis, one of which contained extranodal extension, and one sentinel lymph node was positive with macrometastasis with extranodal capsular involvement.

The patient then began dose-dense adjuvant chemotherapy regimen consisting of Doxorubicin, Cyclophosphamide for initial four cycles and

Paclitaxel for latter four cycles (AC-Pacli) given intravenously once every two weeks for a total of eight treatments.

Staging evaluations including a chest, abdomen, and pelvis CT scans, and bone scan to ensure that there was no distant spread of her disease were performed. The chest CT revealed a well-defined hypodense lesion within the right aspect of the T7 vertebral body measuring 10 mm and was suspicious for metastases. Subsequent MRI showed focal hemangiomas within the spinal vertebrae at T1, T2, T4-T5, T6, T9, T12 and L2 levels, and degenerative changes at multiple levels of the cervical and lumbar spine, with no evidence of vertebral expansion, collapseor significant bony encroachment of the spinal canal or perivertebral soft tissue thickening. The focal lucent area within the T7 vertebral body on the right side showed mild T2 hyperintensity with a peripheral low signal intensity rim and isointense on the T1-weighted image. These findings of the T7 lesion were indeterminate, although its morphology favoured a more benign etiology.

She was then referred to a specialized bone metastases clinic to be seen by a radiation oncologist and an orthopaedic surgeon for further investigation of the suspicious T7 lesion. Upon further review of the imaging of the lesion, it was favoured to be a benign bone hemangioma and not metastases. The patient reported some concern about a recent onset of mild discomfort in her lower back and neck, which was suggestive to be degenerative spine disease, or secondary to her chemotherapy and granulocyte-colony stimulating factor injection. The patient was reassured, and observation and follow-up imaging in three months was recommended. The patient continued with her chemotherapy, and at follow-up one month later was doing well with no symptoms related to her bone hemangiomas.

Literature Review

A literature search was conducted on October 26, 2018 on Ovid Medline (1946 to October Week 2 2018) and Embase (1947 to 2018 week 43). The keywords that were used in this search included 'hemangioma' and 'metastases.' The searches were limited to English language and human subjects only.

Data extraction

Articles were first screened by title and abstract independently by two authors (VR and YR). Potential articles for inclusion were subsequently full-text screened independently by two authors (VR and MMR). A complete description of the screening process can be found in figure 1.

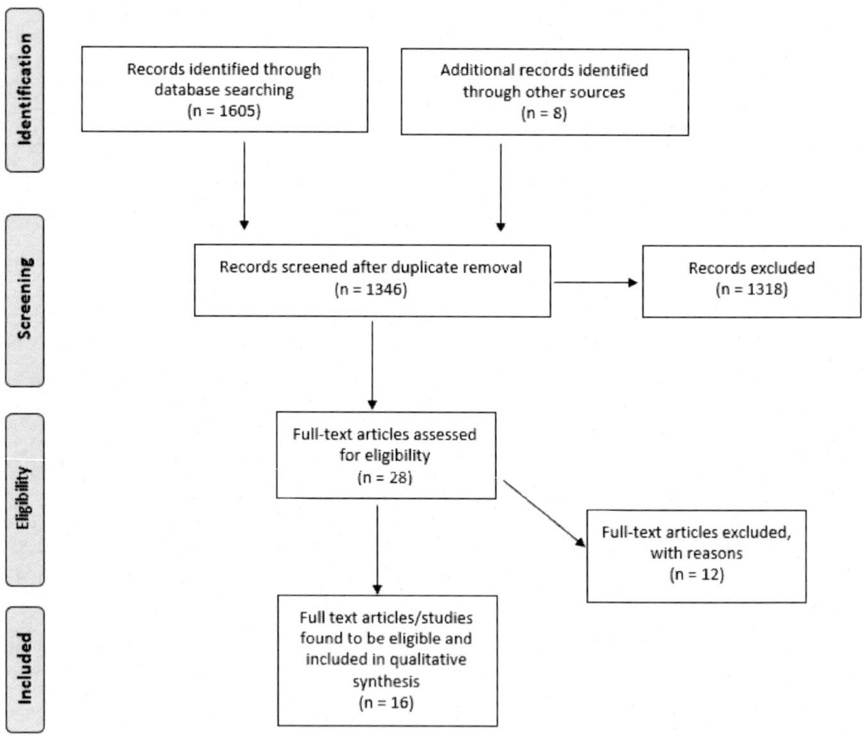

Figure 1. Flowchart of article screening and selection process.

Table 1. Patient characteristics, scan findings, and follow-ups

Author (year)	Age	Sex (M/F)	Cancer type (stage)	Site of bone hemangioma	Size of hemangioma (cm)	Symptoms that led to dx	Relevant scan/ test findings	Tx for hemangioma	Medical history	Medications	FU, number of mos.	Histological subtype
Park, et al. (18)	63	M	None	L 6th rib	5.5 x 2.5 x 1.5	None	**CT**: Osteolytic eccentric expansive mass w/ sunburst calcification and focal cortical disruption at posterolateral arc of L 6th rib; 18F-FDG PET/CT: lesion showed SUV max of 2.4 **Histopathologic analysis of rib**: thin-walled blood vessels w/ dilated channels w/ red blood cells, lined by layer of endothelial cells	Rib resection via postlateral thoracotomy approach	Hyper-tension	Anti-hyperten-sive medication (NS)	x	Caver-nous
Raphael, et al. (3) (case 1)	46	F	Cervix (I)	L1 vertebra	x	Back pain	**Bone scan**: increased tracer uptake in L1 vertebra; **SPECT-CT:** increased tracer uptake in L1 vertebral body; **MRI:** well-defined lesion, hyperintense on T1 and T2-weighted images, multi hypo-intense dots within T2-weighted images; **PET-CT:** no evidence of increased metabolic activity in L1 vertebra lesion, and osteolytic area at L1	x	x	x	FOD, 6	x

Table 1. (Continued)

Author (year)	Age	Sex (M/F)	Cancer type (stage)	Site of bone hemangioma	Size of hemangioma (cm)	Symptoms that led to dx	Relevant scan/ test findings	Tx for hemangioma	Medical history	Medications	FU, number of mos.	Histological subtype
Raphael, et al. (3) (case 2)	54	F	Breast	Multiple vertebral and rib hemangiomas	x	x	**Bone scan**: abnormal increase in tracer uptake in L 2nd rib and thoracolumbar vertebrae; **CT thorax**: multiple hemangiomas of the vertebrae and ribs; **PET-CT**: ruled out skeletal metastases	x	x	x	FOD, 24	x
Manohar, et al. (19)	64	M	Renal cell	D8, L4, D10, L3 vertebrae	x	x	**Bone scintigraphy with MDP:** increased tracer uptake in D8, L4 vertebrae; **SPECT/CT:** MDP uptake in D8 was localized to hemangioma with vertical trabecular thickening on CT, L4 showed MDP avidity with intralesional trabecular thickening, similar lesions seen in D10 and L3 vertebrae; **FDG PET/CT:** no FDG uptake in the lesions, ruling out metastasis	x	x	x	x	x

Author (year)	Age	Sex (M/F)	Cancer type (stage)	Site of bone hemangioma	Size of hemangioma (cm)	Symptoms that led to dx	Relevant scan/ test findings	Tx for hemangioma	Medical history	Medications	FU, number of mos.	Histological subtype
Daoud, et al. (10)	56	F	None	Cervical, thoracic, and lumbar vertebrae, lower sternum, L ischial bone, R iliac crest, L posterior 6th rib, R femoral bone	x	Chronic lower back and neck pain	**Lumbo-sacral X-ray**: osteoblastic lesions in lumbar vertebrae, R iliac crest, and L sacro-iliac joint; **CT pelvis**: areas of increased bone density with surrounding cortical bone destruction in L ischial bone, R iliac crest and L sacro-iliac joint suggesting osteoblastic metastasis; **Tc whole body scan:** multiple bony lesions in cervical, thoracic and lumbar vertebra, lower sternum, L ischial bone, R iliac crest, L posterior 6th rib, R femoral bone suggesting bone metastases; **L pelvic bone biopsy**: sclerosing type of bone hemangioma	Analgesics	Bronchial asthma, micros-copic hematu-ria, osteoporosis	Calcium suppleme-nts, alendronate	Doing well, pain free, no new lesions, 12	x

Table 1. (Continued)

Author (year)	Age	Sex (M/F)	Cancer type (stage)	Site of bone hemangioma	Size of hemangioma (cm)	Symptoms that led to dx	Relevant scan/ test findings	Tx for hemangioma	Medical history	Medications	FU, number of mos.	Histological subtype
Usmani, et al. (17)	66	M	Prostate	D4 vertebra	x	x	**PET-CT:** solitary osteoblastic lesion at D4 vertebral body; **MRI:** features of atypical hemangioma; **Ga-68 PSMA PET-CT:** no signs of bone metastasis; **^{18}F-naF PET-CT** (8-month FU): persistent osteoblastic lesion at D4 without significant change, confirming atypical hemangioma	x	x	x	x	x
Dang et al. (20)	41	F	None	Vertebral body, L pedicles, and lamina of L5, spinal canal, paravertebral region	x	Intermittent back pain for 18 months; numbness of L thoracic wall with intermittent radiating pain; tenderness	**CT:** osteolytic lesion in vertebral body, L pedicles, T5 lamina, disrupted T5 cortex **MRI:** tumor invading entirety of T5 vertebral body, spinal canal and paravertebral region, heterogeneously hypointense on T1-weighted image and	Combined laminectomy + vertebraplasty; excision of the epidural soft tumor mass; postoperative RT 30Gy 4 weeks after surgery	x	x	x	x

Author (year)	Age	Sex (M/F)	Cancer type (stage)	Site of bone hemangioma	Size of hemangioma (cm)	Symptoms that led to dx	Relevant scan/ test findings	Tx for hemangioma	Medical history	Medications	FU, number of mos.	Histological subtype
						along middle thoracic spine	hyperintense on T2-weighted image, significant increase in signal intensity; **MRI:** compression of dural sac by epidural extension of tumor; **PET-CT:** T5 lesion, SUV of 1.3 Biopsy of paravertebral lesion: distinct histopathological diagnosis of vertebral hemangioma					
Shi et al. (21)	60	F	None	Tll vertebra	x	x	Isointense signal lesion at T11-vertebrae on T1-weighted image; isointense signal of fat supressed T1-weighted images; **CT:** hypo-dense lesion with internal striated appearance	x	x	x	x	

Table 1. (Continued)

Author (year)	Age	Sex (M/F)	Cancer type (stage)	Site of bone hemangioma	Size of hemangioma (cm)	Symptoms that led to dx	Relevant scan/ test findings	Tx for hemangioma	Medical history	Medications	FU, number of mos.	Histological subtype
Ching et al. (14)	52	F	None	L knee	x	L lower limb pain for several years; L knee pain leading to impaired mobility; weight loss	**Radiograph:** isodense lesion to the bone located within the medullary cavity, with a sclerotic margin at epiphysis of proximal tibia and lesion with central lucency with a; sclerotic margin at the diaphysis of L femur and proximal L fibula **Surgical biopsy w/ osteotomy of L mid fibula:** thin-walled blood vessels w/ ad-jacent bony trabeculae, vascular channels of dilated venous-calibre type and capillary sized vessels, no malignant cells	Open biopsy w/ segmental osteotomy	Stage I membrane-ous nephron-pathy; hyper-tension	Yes / treated symptomatic ally(NS)	Pain free, 12	Mixed capillary and venous

Author (year)	Age	Sex (M/F)	Cancer type (stage)	Site of bone hemangioma	Size of hemangioma (cm)	Symptoms that led to dx	Relevant scan/ test findings	Tx for hemangioma	Medical history	Medications	FU, number of mos.	Histological subtype
Lakemeier, et al. (22)	44	F	None	C7 vertebra	x	Paresthesia in forearms + hands for 3 months; pain + paresthesia in face	**X-ray:** osteolysis of C7 vertebra; **MRI:** increased signal intensity on T2-weighted images, diagnosis of metastatic osteolysis of C7 was made; **Intensive immune-histochemical work-up:** distinct vascularization of lesion with partially collapsed sinusoidal and slit-like blood vessels, no cytologic atypia or increased mitotic rate were seen, hemangioma with reactive osteoid formation was made	Corporectomy of C7; implantation of customary titanium cage	None	x	Pain free cervical spine movement, loss of rotation of 20 degrees, normal alignment of spine, 6	Capillary

Table 1. (Continued)

Author (year)	Age	Sex (M/F)	Cancer type (stage)	Site of bone hemangioma	Size of hemangioma (cm)	Symptoms that led to dx	Relevant scan/ test findings	Tx for hemangioma	Medical history	Medications	FU, number of mos.	Histological subtype
Wallis et al. (23)	52	F	None	Iliac crest; dorsal and lumbosacral spine; ribs; skull	x	7 year history of dull, sharp, shooting back pain, radiating in a bilateral radicular distribu-tion, around lower thorax, abdomen, and hips, thighs, knees, legs and ankles	**Roentgenograms of chest:** extensive metastases in the lungs, osteoblastic and osteolytic metastases in the skull, pelvis, spine, and long bones, lytic lesions in both ilia; **Thyroidectomy:** nodular goiter and no evidence of carcinoma, ruling out the thyroid as the primary source of metastases; **Lung biopsy:** nodular fibrosis of unknown etiology; **Rib biopsy:** normal bone and skeletal muscle; **Iliac biopsy**: mixed	1000 calorie diet; exercise regimen; thyroid replacement; dextropropoxyphene; 2700 cGy to lumbar spine	Hemorrhoids caused by constipation, chronic cigarette cough, obesity, hard nodule on thyroid	x	Mild occasi-onal backa-ches, NS	Mixed capillary and cavernous

Author (year)	Age	Sex (M/F)	Cancer type (stage)	Site of bone hemangioma	Size of hemangioma (cm)	Symptoms that led to dx	Relevant scan/ test findings	Tx for hemangioma	Medical history	Medications	FU, number of mos.	Histological subtype
							capillary and cavernous hemangioma of the bone					
Leeds et al. (15)	40	x	Ocular mela-noma; hepatic metasta-sis	L2 vertebral body	x	x	**MRI:** abnormal increase in sagittal T1-weighted signal intensity of lesion, decrease in signal intensity on sagittal FSE T2-weighted, fat-suppressed image, intense enhancement on postcontrast sagittal T1 weighted, fat-suppressed image; **CT:** A sharply defined lesion with trabecular pattern **MRI:** A sharply defined lesion with low signal intensity on T1-weighted image, high signal	x	x	x	x	x

Table 1. (Continued)

Author (year)	Age	Sex (M/F)	Cancer type (stage)	Site of bone hemangioma	Size of hemangioma (cm)	Symptoms that led to dx	Relevant scan/ test findings	Tx for hemangioma	Medical history	Medications	FU, number of mos.	Histological subtype
Leeds et al. (15)	x	x	x	L3 vertebral body	x	x	intensity on T2 with fat suppression and homogeneous intense enhancement on post-contrast sagittal T1 fat-suppressed image; **Axial post-contrast T1-weighted MRI:** prominent basi-vertebral plexus, draining from the hemangioma, distinct vascular channel	x	x	x	x	x
Laguna et al. (24)	62	M	Papillary thyroid carcinoma with metastases to cervical nodes	T5 vertebra	x	None	**Whole-body I-131 scan**: abnormal focal area of I-131 tracer concentration in the chest; **CT spine:** dense trabecular pattern in the vertebral body resembling a hemangioma	x	x	x	Symptom free, NS	x

Author (year)	Age	Sex (M/F)	Cancer type (stage)	Site of bone hemangioma	Size of hemangioma (cm)	Symptoms that led to dx	Relevant scan/ test findings	Tx for hemangioma	Medical history	Medications	FU, number of mos.	Histological subtype
Zito et al. (11)	58	M	x	Skull, T2, T3, T6, T9, T10, L4, T6, sacrum	x	Bilateral leg weakness; difficulty walking; occasional falls; burning pain in the back and legs; a band-like sensation around the mid-thorax; urinary urgency; incomplete bladder emptying; constipa-tion	**X-ray of spine and pelvis:** lucent areas with parallel vertical striations in T2, T3, T6, T9, T10, L4, and L5 bodies, similar lesion in the R superior sacrum, paravertebral mass in the midthoracic region, oval radiolucent lesion in the L frontal bone w/honeycomb like appearance; **Myelography:** compressive lesion blocking upward flow at T6 and downward flow at T2; **Spinal angiography:** vascular lesions at T6 & T10, w/prominent extraosseous staining; **Biopsy of T2 vertebrae:** capillary hemangioma	Intravenous dexamethasone therapy, and a decompre-ssive laminectomy was performed from T2 to T6	x	Intravenous dexamethasone therapy, decompressive lami-nectomy from T2 to T6	No neurolo-gical abnor-malities except mild proximal leg weakn-ess and hyper-reflexia	Capillary

Table 1. (Continued)

Author (year)	Age	Sex (M/F)	Cancer type (stage)	Site of bone hemangioma	Size of hemangioma (cm)	Symptoms that led to dx	Relevant scan/ test findings	Tx for hemangioma	Medical history	Medications	FU, number of mos.	Histological subtype
Kulsh-restha et al. (25)	45	M	None	T1 vertebra; R 9th rib; L 8th rib	x	Coldness, numbness and clumsiness in the legs; exacerbated by neck flexion or hand use, which caused "pins and needles" or electric shocks to go down the backs of his legs to the soles of his feet	**Thyroid scan:** increased uptake in one lobe, appearing to be a benign adenoma; **Bone scan**: increased uptake at T1, R 9th rib, 10th rib; **MRI:** increase in signal intensity on T2 weighted images, as well as mottled appearance of T1 vertebral body. This was reported as metastatic disease; **Vertebrectomy:** when attempted, caused massive arterial bleeding from the bone, thus only partial removal of T1 body was possible;	Vertebrec-tomy for neural decompress-sion (prior to hemangioma diagnosis); embolization therapy via a branch of T5 intercostal artery	Appendectomy; sponta-neous pneumothorax	x	Symp-tom-free	x

Author (year)	
Age	
Sex (M/F)	
Cancer type (stage)	
Site of bone hemangioma	
Size of hemangioma (cm)	
Symptoms that led to dx	
Relevant scan/ test findings	**Histopathological analysis of bone removed from vertebrectomy:** wide thin-walled blood-filled spaces and sinuses lined by endothelium interspersed among trabeculae of bone, typical of bone hemangioma; **CT of T1:** revealed vertebral hemangioma; **CT of L 8th and R 9th ribs:** vertical trabeculae, consistent with bone hemangioma
Tx for hemangioma	
Medical history	
Medications	
FU, number of mos.	
Histological subtype	

Table 1. (Continued)

Author (year)	Age	Sex (M/F)	Cancer type (stage)	Site of bone hemangioma	Size of hemangioma (cm)	Symptoms that led to dx	Relevant scan/ test findings	Tx for hemangioma	Medical history	Medications	FU, number of mos.	Histological subtype
Puri et al. (26)	63	M	None	4th rib	6.5x5x2.5	L chest wall pain; dyspnea	**X-ray chest:** radiopaque shadow in L mid and lower zone; **Contrast enhanced CT:** heterogenous, expansile, osteolytic, eccentric bony outgrowth at 4th rib; histopathological examination of rib: encapsulated, globular, expansible lesion which measured 6.5x5x2.5 cm in size, cut surface showed cystic degeneration filled with hemorrhage, dilated and congested thin and thick-walled vascular spaces, bony trabeculae lined by conspicuous	x	x	x	x	x

Author (year)	Age	Sex (M/F)	Cancer type (stage)	Site of bone hemangioma	Size of hemangioma (cm)	Symptoms that led to dx	Relevant scan/ test findings	Tx for hemangioma	Medical history	Medications	FU, number of mos.	Histological subtype
							osteoblastic rimming present, diagnosed as hemangioma					
Bellasri et al. (27)	40	F	None	T7 vertebrae		Dorsal pain; weakness and numbness in lower limbs; Upgoing toes bilaterally; bilateral patellar tendon hyperre-flexia	**MRI:** T7 expansile bone mass involving spine, low T1 signal intensity, heterogeneous high T2 signal intensity; **Surgery with posterior approach:** highly vascularized lesion; **Histologic analysis:** numerous think walled vascular channels in collagenous connective tissue, with single layer of endothelial cells, hemangioma diagnosis made	Complete resection of tumor	x	x	No pain or weak-ness; walking with normal posture; signify-cant spinal cord decompre ssion,1-week post-op; 4 weeks; 2 months	Cavernous

Table 1. (Continued)

Author (year)	Age	Sex (M/F)	Cancer type (stage)	Site of bone hemangioma	Size of hemangioma (cm)	Symptoms that led to dx	Relevant scan/ test findings	Tx for hemangioma	Medical history	Medications	FU, number of mos.	Histological subtype
Rico et al. (present case)	50	F	Breast	T1, T2, T4, T5, T6, T7, T9, T12, L2 vertebrae	T7: 10mm	None	**Chest CT:** well-defined hypodensity with R aspect of T7 vertebral body; **MRI:** focal hemangiomas within spinal vertebrae at T1, T2, T4, T5, T6, T9, T12, L2	None	x	x	Symptom free, 1	x

M, male; F, female; Tx, treatment; SUV max, maximum standardized uptake value; CT, Computed Tomography; NS, not specified; BS, bone scan; RT, radiation therapy; MDP, methylene diphosphate; FDG, fluorodeoxyglucose; PET, positron emission tomography; SPECT, single photon emission computed tomography; L, left; R, right; Mets, metastasis; MRI, magnetic resonance imaging; Ga-68 PSMA, Gallium-68-prostate-specific membrane antigen; 18F-naF PET-CT, 18F-sodium fluoride positron emission tomography-computed tomography; FOD, free of disease; NS, not specified.

Articles met the inclusion criteria for this review if they described cases that reported on hemangiomas of the bone or where an incorrect diagnosis or speculation of metastases instead of hemangioma was originally made. The exclusion criteria for this review included: i) hemangiomas located in places other than the bone, ii) hemangiomas where potential metastasis was not considered during the diagnostic process, iii) articles that did not report information on individual cases. Non-original articles, including reviews and editorials were also excluded.

Available information on patient characteristics, medical histories, hemangioma characteristics, scan or test results, medications, treatments, and follow-up outcomes were extracted by two authors (VR and MMR) and can be found in Table 1.

SEARCH RESULTS

The literature search generated a total of 1,605 articles: 1,210 from Embase, and 395 from Ovid Medline. A total of 24 articles were included for full text screening. Of the 24 articles that were full-text screened, 16 articles met the inclusion criteria for this review (3, 8-22). Table 1 contains a summary of the reviewed articles, including patient characteristics, relevant scans and tests and patient-reported symptoms.

Patient characteristics

This literature review summarizes 19 cases of bone hemangiomas that resembled or were initially misdiagnosed as bone metastases (3, 8-22). Eighteen of 19 cases reported age, and the average age across these 18 cases was 56.6 years and ranged from 40 to 66 years old. Sex was reported in 17 of 19 cases (89.5%), with 7 of 17 cases being male patients (41.2%), and 10 of 17 cases being female patients (58.8%) (3, 8, 10-22).

In 12 of 19 cases (63.2%), it was stated that the patient either did not have cancer, or there was no primary cancer reported; thus, we assumed that they did not have cancer (10, 11, 14, 15, 18, 20–23, 25-27). Among the seven patients that reported a primary cancer, the most common site was the breast (n = 2, 10.5%).

Ten of 19 hemangioma cases (52.6%) occurred solely in the spinal or vertebral region, and five cases (26.3%) featured multiple hemangiomas of the spinal or vertebral region, in addition to other bony sites; thus, 15 of 19 cases (79.0%) had vertebral or spinal hemangiomas (3, 11, 15, 17, 19–27). Two of 19 cases (10.5%) reported on hemangiomas occurring in the rib alone, while four cases (21.1%) reported on rib hemangiomas in addition to hemangiomas in other bone regions; thus, a total of six cases reported on hemangiomas of the rib (31.6%) (3, 10, 18, 23, 25, 26). Two cases reported on hemangiomas of the skull in addition to other bone regions (10.5%) (11,23). Other regions that bone hemangiomas were found are summarized in table 1.

Nine of 19 cases (47.4%) either reported that the patient had no symptoms associated with the bone hemangioma, or no symptoms were described; thus, we assumed they were asymptomatic (3, 15, 17–19, 21, 24). Ten of 19 patients (52.6%) reported at least one symptom, such as back pain (n=5, 50.0%) or leg weakness and numbness (n=3, 30.0%) in patients presenting with vertebral hemangiomas (3, 10, 11, 14, 20, 22, 23, 25, 27). One patient (10.0%) with a rib hemangioma reported chest wall pain (26). One patient (10.0%) with a cervical vertebral hemangioma reported paresthesia in her forearms and hands, as well as pain and paresthesia in her face (22). Another patient (10.0%) with a knee hemangioma reported pain in her lower limb and knee area (14). Additional symptoms reported by patients are described in table 1.

Nine of 19 patients (47.4%) underwent some type of treatment or intervention for their bone hemangioma (3, 10, 11, 14, 15, 17–21, 23-27) described in greater detail in Table 1. Of note, not all patients who received intervention presented with symptoms, as some of these interventions were done to aid in the diagnosis of the bone hemangioma, rather than treat symptoms associated with the hemangioma.

Histological subtype data was only available for five of 19 patients (26.3%) (14, 18, 22, 27, 28). Of these five patients, two were cavernous

(40.0%) (18, 27), one was capillary (20.0%) (22), one was mixed capillary and cavernous (20.0%) (23), and one was mixed capillary and venous (20.0%) (14).

Follow-up information was available for 11 of 19 patients (57.9%) (3, 10, 11, 14, 22–25, 27). Two of 19 (10.5%) patients were free-of-disease at follow-up (3). Seven of 19 patients (36.8%) were symptom or pain-free at follow-up (10, 14, 22, 24, 25, 27). One patient (5.3%) reported mild, occasional back pain at follow-up (23). One patient (5.3%) reported no neurological abnormalities but had proximal leg weakness and hyperreflexia at follow–up (11).

CONCLUSION AND DISCUSSION

Diagnosing bone hemangiomas can be difficult when they appear as atypical upon medical imaging. Bone hemangiomas that are mistakenly diagnosed as bone metastases can lead to additional anxiety and worry for patients and family members and non-essential tests and imaging (29). Determining effective diagnostic strategies to differentiate hemangiomas and metastases should be a target for future investigation. Additionally, determining treatment protocol and management of bone hemangiomas should be a focus of study in the future.

Bone hemangiomas are rare, and most commonly occur in the vertebrae and skull (2). Large autopsy studies and radiographic scan reviews have concluded that hemangiomas are the most common benign lesions found in the spine, with an approximate incidence of 10-12% within the general population (30). After reviewing the literature, 15 of 19 cases (79.0%) involved vertebral or spinal hemangiomas mistaken for metastases, while only two of 19 cases (10.5%) involved hemangiomas of the skull mistaken for metastases. This may suggest that despite being a common type of hemangioma, skull hemangiomas may present with a more typical appearance on radiographic imaging than vertebral hemangiomas, resulting in less frequent confusion with metastases.

When hemangiomas appear as atypical, many of the classic characteristics of hemangiomas that aid in their diagnosis are not present (14). MRI is regarded as the imaging modality that provides the clearest description of hemangiomas (10). However, MRI intensities of atypical hemangiomas may not lead to a direct diagnosis of hemangioma, and thus, examining the morphology of the lesion may help aid in making an accurate diagnosis. CT scans may be used in these cases, since they have a higher sensitivity for detecting bone remodeling (17). While diagnosis of bone hemangiomas is frequently accomplished based on radiographic appearance of the hemangioma, in atypical hemangioma cases a bone biopsy is warranted to differentiate from metastasis, cysts or other bony lesions (31). To illustrate the challenges with atypical hemangiomas, Ching et al. noted that typical hemangiomas of non-spinal sites are radiolucent, expansile and are distinct with a radiating type pattern; however, one of their hemangioma cases was found to have both lucent and isodense areas, with reactive sclerotic margins, suggestive of osteoid osteoma (14). Moreover, Ching et al. (14) described another case where on CT scan, a vertebral hemangioma appeared to have ring-shaped lucencies with sclerotic rings, which differs from the typical polka-dot appearance of vertebral body hemangiomas (14).

Bone hemangiomas are often found incidentally on scanning assessments due to their asymptomatic tendencies. Including the reviewed cases and the case from our centre, nine of 19 cases (47.4%) had no reported symptoms associated with their bone hemangioma (3, 15, 17–19, 21, 24). It is important to note that symptomatic patients may have been experiencing such symptoms as a result of their cancer, and not necessarily because of the hemangioma itself. A study that examined 59 cases of vertebral hemangiomas from 1980 to 1990 found 35 (59.3%) of these hemangiomas incidentally, and 13 of them (22.0%) due to associated pain. This study highlighted the asymptomatic nature of bone hemangiomas and noted that they are often found incidentally.

Given that hemangiomas are often asymptomatic in nature, they commonly do not require medical intervention or treatment. However, in cases where hemangiomas are more aggressive, they may require treatment. Although rare, some vertebral hemangiomas may act aggressively and invade the paravertebral space or spinal canal, resulting in potential compression of the spinal cord or nerve roots (30). Occurrence of such compressions are seen most commonly in hemangiomas of the thoracic spine (30). There is no clear consensus among health care providers on the standard treatment protocol for aggressive hemangiomas and thus, these concepts should be further explored.

Fox et al. (30) historically reviewed 11 patients with vertebral hemangiomas with spinal cord compression. All 11 patients initially underwent decompressive surgery and had complete neurological recovery. Six patients underwent subtotal tumor resection and subsequent radiation therapy (RT) of 1000 cGy or less; of which three patients (50.0%) had recurrent neurological symptoms. All four patients who underwent subtotal tumor resection plus RT had no recurrences. One patient who underwent gross tumor resection did not recur when examined at follow-up of an unspecified time period. These patient findings and a review of the literature led the authors of this article to recommend yearly neurological and radiological examination in patients with painful hemangiomas, and stated that this is particularly important for young females with thoracic hemangiomas. RT and embolization are also effective treatments for individuals with moderate to severe constant pain. The authors state that those with asymptomatic hemangiomas do not require regular follow-up, unless pain corresponding to the hemangioma develops. The authors conclude that patients with neurological deficits should undergo preoperative embolization and angiography, decompressive surgery, and RT in patients who undergo subtotal tumor resection (30).

Uncertainty surrounding imaging methods for bone hemangiomas remain a clinical challenge and determining the best detection methods for these lesions should be the focus of future investigation. Forming a consensus for treatment protocols of bone hemangiomas should be another target for studies. Bone hemangiomas, especially those that are atypical in appearance, may lead to diagnostic and treatment uncertainty. In such cases where lesions are equivocal or indeterminate, a radiologist should be consulted to proceed with a diagnosis and treatment plan.

ACKNOWLEDGEMENTS

We thank the generous support of Bratty Family Fund, Michael and Karyn Goldstein Cancer Research Fund, Joey and Mary Furfari Cancer Research Fund, Pulenzas Cancer Research Fund, Joseph and Silvana Melara Cancer Research Fund, and Ofelia Cancer Research Fund. The authors declare that there is no conflict of interest. Written consent was obtained from the patient to allow for the publication of this report and any relevant accompanying images.

REFERENCES

[1] Pack GT, Miller TR. Hemangiomas: Classification, diagnosis and treatment. Angiology 1950;1(5):405–26.

[2] Dorfman HD, Steinel GC, Jaffe HL. Vascular tumors of the bone. Hum Pathol 1971;2(3):349–76.

[3] Raphael J, Hephzibah J, Mani S, Shanthly N, Oommen R. Abnormal appearance of spinal hemangioma mimicking metastasis in bone scintigraphy and SPECT-CT: Case report. J Nucl Med Radiat Ther 2013;S6(016):1–3.

[4] Rokan Z, Kealey WD. Osteomalacia: A forgotten cause of fractures in the elderly. BMJ Case Rep 2015;2015:1–2. doi: 10.1136/bcr-2014-207184.

[5] McCarthy EF, Frassica FJ. Pathology of bone and joint disorders with clinical and radiographic correlation. Cambridge: Cambridge University Press, 2014.

[6] Aksu G, Fayda M, Saynak M, Karadeniz A. Spinal cord compression due to vertebral hemangioma. Orthopedics 2008;31(2):169.

[7] Heindel W, Gübitz R, Vieth V, Weckesser M, Schober O, Schäfers M. The diagnostic imaging of bone metastases. Dtsch Arztebl Int 2014;111(44):741–7.

[8] Morales KA, Arevalo-Perez J, Holodny AI, Lis E, Karimi S. Differentiating atypical hemangiomas and metastatic vertebral lesions? The role of T1-weighted dynamic. Am Soc Neuroradiol 2018;39(5):968-73.

[9] Rodallec MH, Feydy A, Larousserie F, Anract P, Campagna R, Babinet A, et al. Diagnostic imaging of solitary tumors of the spine: What to do and say. Radiographics 2008;28(4):1019–41.

[10] Daoud E. Multiple bone hemangiomas presenting as bony metastasis of unknown primary. J Med 2010;11(2):196–9.

[11] Zito G, Kadis GN. Multiple vertebral hemangiomas resembling metastases with spinal cord compression. Arch Neurol 1980;37(4):247–8.

[12] Ross JS, Masaryk TJ, Modic MT, Carter JR, Mapstone T, Dengel FH. Vertebral hemangiomas: MR imaging. Radiology 1987;165(1):165–9.

[13] Gaudino S, Martucci M, Colantonio R, Lozupone E, Visconti E, Leone A, et al. A systematic approach to vertebral hemangioma. Skeletal Radiol 2015;44(1):25–36.

[14] Ching BC, Wong JSL, Tan MH, Jara-lazaro AR. The many faces of intraosseous haemangioma: A diagnostic headache. Singapore Med J 2009;50(5):195–8.

[15] Leeds NE, Kumar A, Zhou XJ, McKinnon GC. Magnetic resonance imaging of benign spinal lesions simulating metastasis: Role of diffusion-weighted imaging. Top Magn Reson Imaging 2000;11(4):224–34.

[16] Cross JJ, Antoun NM, Laing RJC, Xuereb J. Imaging of compressive vertebral haemangiomas. Eur Radiol 2000;10(6):997–1002.

[17] Usmani S, Marafi F, Rasheed R, Al Kandari F, Ahmed N. Atypical hemangioma mimicking metastasis on 18F-sodium fluoride positron emission tomography-computed tomography and magnetic resonance imaging: Gallium-68-prostate-specific membrane antigen positron emission tompgraphy improves the specificity of bone lesions. Indian J Nucl Med 2018;33(2):171–3.

[18] Park JY, Gyoon PJ, Lee SJ. Cavernous hemangioma of the breast: A case report. Iran J Radiol 2016;13(3):1–3.

[19] Manohar K, Paraghane R, Kumari S, Bhattacharya A, Mandal A, Mittal B. Multiple vertebral hemangiomas mimicking metastases in a patient with renal carcinoma: Importance of hybrid imaging with SPECT/CT and FDG PET/CT. J Postgrad Med 2012;46(4):196–7.

[20] Dang L, Liu C, Yang SM, Jiang L, Liu ZJ, Liu XG, et al. Aggressive vertebral hemangioma of the thoracic spine without typical radiological appearance. Eur Spine J 2012;21(10):1994–9.

[21] Shi Y-J, Li X-T, Zhang X-Y, Liu Y-L, Tang L, Sun Y-S. Differential diagnosis of hemangiomas from spinal osteolytic metastases using 3.0 T MRI: Comparison of T1-weighted imaging, chemical-shift imaging, diffusion-weighted and contrast-enhanced imaging. Oncotarget 2017;8(41):71095–104.

[22] Lakemeier S, Westhoff CC, Fuchs-Winkelmann S, Schofer MD. Osseous hemangioma of the seventh cervical vertebra with osteoid formation mimicking metastasis: A case report. J Med Case Rep 2009;3(92):1–4.

[23] Wallis LA, Asch T, Maisel BW. Diffuse skeletal hemangiomatosis: report of two cases and review of literature. Am J Med 1964;37(4):545–63.

[24] Laguna R, Silva F, Vazquez-Selles J, Orduna E, Flores C. Vertebral hemangioma mimicking a metastatic bone lesion in well-differentiated thyroid carcinoma. Clin Nucl Med 2000;25(8):611–3.

[25] Kulshrestha M, Byrne P. Multiple primary haemangiomas of bone mimicking vertebral metastases. J R Soc Med 1997;90(11):632–4.

[26] Puri S, Gupta N, Asotra S. Hemangioma of rib masquerading a malignancy. J Cancer Res Ther 2018;14(10):809–11.

[27] Bellasri S, Fatihi J, Elktaibi A, El Asri A. Acute spinal cord compression caused by atypical vertebral hemangioma. J Craniovertebr Junction Spine 2017;8(3):275.

[28] Wallis LA, Asch T, Maisel BW. Diffuse skeletal hemangiomatosis. Am J Med 1964;37:545–63.

[29] Scolyer RA, Zhuang L, Palmer AA, Thompson JF, McCarthy SW. Combined naevus: A benign lesion frequently misdiagnosed both clinically and pathologically as melanoma. Pathology 2004;36(5):419–27.

[30] Fox MW, Onofrio BM. The natural history and management of symptomatic and asymptomatic vertebral hemangiomas. J Neurosurg 1993;78(1):36–45.

[31] Huvos A. Bone tumors: Diagnosis, treatment and prognosis, 2nd ed. Philadelphia, PA: WB Saunders, 1987.

In: Pain Management
Editors: J Merrick and M Morad
ISBN: 978-1-68507-493-7

Chapter 20

EMOTIONAL PAIN OR PHYSICAL PAIN: THE CONTRIBUTION OF HEDONICS IN MOTOR PERFORMANCE OF ATHLETES?

Mahboubeh Ghayour Najafabadi*, PhD
and Amirhossein Memari, MD
Department of Motor Behavior, Faculty of Physical Education
University of Tehran, Tehran and Sports Medicine Research Center,
Neuroscience Institute, Tehran University of Medical Sciences,
Tehran, Iran

ABSTRACT

Examining of athletes who have maladaptive hedonics including physical or emotional displeasure or pain is very important in sports. Indeed, the aim of this case study was to compare the balance ability of three volleyball athletes in two conditions inducing physical pain or emotional pain. We designed two kinds of induced pain and assessed balance in

* ***Correspondence:*** Mahboubeh Ghayour Najafabadi, Department of Physical Education and Sport Sciences, University of Tehran, North Kargar Avenue, Amirabad Street, Tehran. Email: m.ghayournaj@ut.ac.ir.

these expert athletes in medio-lateral index (MLI), anterior posterior index (API) and overall balance. The results showed that API and overall balance scores have largely increased from baseline to physical or emotional pain condition while MLI score showed different pattern. In total, an athlete under emotional pain condition would experience same disturbance in balance scores as physical pain condition.

INTRODUCTION

In addition to physiological (for example stress) and biomechanical (for example technique), psychological factors also play a crucial role in sport performance (1, 2). Although there is a consensus on deteriorating effects of physical stress or pain on athletes' performance (3), we are not aware of effects of social or emotional pain as psychological factors on performance of athletes. The 'emotional pain' is defined as the unpleasant experience associated with actual or potential damage to one's sense of social connection or emotional value (owing to be socially stressed or observing the others in emotionally adverse conditions) (4). For example, in competition, athletes have often heard phrases such as "you are a failure" or "you were not able to receive this ball" that implies socially disconnecting experiences. In the current study we tried to examine athletes who have maladaptive hedonics including physical or emotional displeasure or pain. Indeed, the aim of this case study was to compare the balance ability of three volleyball athletes in two conditions inducing physical pain or emotional pain.

CASES

Three elite volleyball players (20-25 year-old female) were referred to a clinic of sports medicine due to performance related complaints. The athletes reported poor performance during competition with spectators, but not in training sessions or matches without any spectators. All had sport experiences for 10 to 12 years. Furthermore they had no active sport injury during the study time.

We used Biodex system for assessing balance of athletes; and medio-lateral index (MLI), anterior posterior index (API) and overall balance scores. We also administered VAS (a 10-cm horizontal line) for getting the rate of emotional and physical pain. For assessing a base of balance, the athletes dressed with sport clothing and stood in the center of the platform in a stable position. We then used an algometer for inducing pain in three trials with 30-second rest intervals. Induction of pain on tibial crest was performed by Commander Algometer (JTECH Medical, UT, USA). The recommended point was two cm away in the midline of the tibial crest that was marked with a surgical pen to keep constant positions for all observations. The pressure was given until the participants reported a significant increase of pain or discomfort. After two days, the emotional pain task was designed on the basis of showing images related to sport injury while participants standing on the platform. Images were showed in distance of two meters from participants three times with 30 seconds rest intervals.

Furthermore athletes were assessed for physical or emotional pain by VAS; finally we analyzed those trials with the same score in VAS for physical and emotional pain (5). All participants gave informed consent and the study was approved by the Institutional Ethics Committee.

FINDINGS

In all cases, anterior posterior index (API) and overall balance scores increased from baseline to physical or emotional pain condition, while medio-lateral index (MLI) score showed different pattern (see Figure 1). Although there were differences in patterns of balance scores among three athletes; the general trend of changes from baseline to pain conditions are comparable at least in graphical presentations. In other words, athletes under emotional pain condition would experience same disturbance in balance scores as physical pain condition.

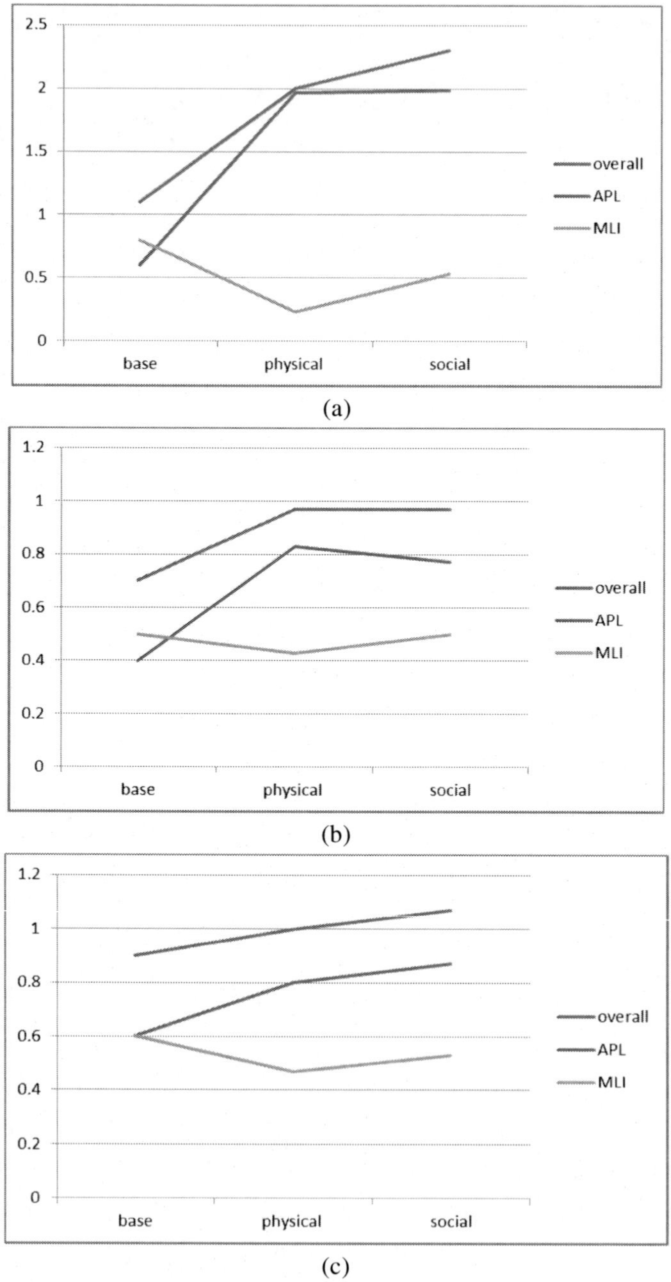

Figure 1. Case 1 (a): 11 years of experience in volleyball; Case 2 (b): 12 years of experience in volleyball and case 3 (c): 10 years of experience of volleyball.

CONCLUSION AND DISCUSSION

Reflect on two sport scenarios; in the first scenario, during a competition, you have muscle injury or a sprained leg with an experience of severe pain. In the second scenario, you just look at pictures of athletes with sport-related injuries; the same as you look at pictures, you suffer from emotional discomfort and feel another class of pain. Our preliminary observation from these two scenarios showed that to some extent, experiences of emotional pain and physical pain in athletes might be comparable. As far as we know, this is the first time to report that both emotional pain and physical pain influenced athletes motor function (6).

Although there is a consensus that athletes can tolerate pain better than other people (7), athletes are regularly confronted with physically as well as socially or emotionally challenging situations. Consequently, athletes frequently experience persistent pain or pressure in field or off field (8). On the other side, the performance of important motor tasks (e.g., postural control) is part of the training and competition practice in sports, such as for example volleyball in which pain may affect the physical or psychological performance of the athletes.

Studies on physical pain confirmed that either low back pain in athletes or even patellar tendinopathy in non-athletes would impair postural control; in fact those with pain used higher level of energy with larger sway amplitude to control postural stability (9, 10). However there is some research that could not replicate the previous studies and suggested no association between back pain of athletes and postural control (11, 12).

Addressing the novelty of our study, stress and emotional pain is a complex and ubiquitous experience for athletes. A few peripheral variables manipulate an athlete's experience of pain, for example opponents or fans aggression, their failures or unfavorable injury scenes. These pressures involve the athlete's mental and physical resources (e.g., mental skills, motor control) (13). For example postural control impairment could be a consequent pain response on an interaction level among emotional, social, and motor systems (8).

To address the, the overlap between neural mechanisms underlying the experience of emotional pain and physical pain as an adaptive neuroevolutionary strategy was suggested as a possible mechanism of observed findings. There are the common brain regions for example the dACC and AI that may contribute to inflammatory activity due to physical or emotional pain. In turn, increases in inflammatory activity following emotional and physical pain could impair immune system function and destroys cognitive performance and motor function in elite athletes (14, 15).

Our current results can extend the future research on socio-emotional and physical pain in sport context in order to examine athletes' performance as well as share representation in somatosensory brain networks. Other researchers may be interested to identify other source of athletes' distress during competitions and their consequences (16). In consequence, and as an implication for practice, sport clinician or sport psychologist can use specific interventions for managing emotional pain in athletes who may show poor performance during competition (17).

This finding should be considered in a context of a case report research; however a limitation of the present study is how to generate physical or emotional pain. Inducing emotional pain in athletes needs more sophisticated future methodology, in order to enhance ecological validity of experimenting emotional pain and athletes' performance.

ACKNOWLEDGMENT

We want to thank the athletes who participated in the study. This study was supported by University of Tehran (Grant number: 30701.1.1)

REFERENCES

[1] Bali A. Psychological factors affecting sports performance. Intern J Phys Educ Sports Health 2015;1(6):92-5.

[2] Alizadeh R, Shariat A, Nakhostin Ansari N, Kordi R, Cleland JA, Hakakzad A, et al. Office-based exercise therapy as a non-pharmacological treatment for discogenic low back pain among army staff. Iran J Public Health 2018;47(12):1969-70.

[3] Hainline B, Turner JA, Caneiro J, Stewart M, Moseley GL. Pain in elite athletes-neurophysiological, biomechanical and psychosocial considerations: A narrative review. Br J Sports Med 2017;51(17):1259-64.

[4] Eisenberger NI. The pain of social disconnection: examining the shared neural underpinnings of physical and social pain. Nat Rev Neurosci 2012;13(6):421.

[5] DeWall CN, Baumeister RF. Alone but feeling no pain: Effects of social exclusion on physical pain tolerance and pain threshold, affective forecasting, and interpersonal empathy. J Pers Soc Psychol 2006;91(1):1.

[6] Chen S, Jackson T. Causal effects of challenge and threat appraisals on pain self-efficacy, pain coping, and tolerance for laboratory pain: An experimental path analysis study. PloS One 2019;14(4):e0215087.

[7] Deroche T, Woodman T, Stephan Y, Brewer BW, Le Scanff C. Athletes' inclination to play through pain: a coping perspective. Anxiety Stress Coping 2011;24(5):579-87.

[8] Heidari J, Mierswa T, Kleinert J, Ott I, Levenig C, Hasenbring M, et al. Parameters of low back pain chronicity among athletes: Associations with physical and mental stress. Phys Ther Sport 2016;21:31-7.

[9] Rosen AB, Ko J, Brown CN. The relationship between acute pain and dynamic postural stability indices in individuals with patellar tendinopathy. Gait Posture 2018;65:117-20.

[10] Oyarzo CA, Villagran CR, Silvestre RE, Carpintero P, Berral FJ. Postural control and low back pain in elite athletes comparison of static balance in elite athletes with and without low back pain. J Back Musculoskelet Rehabil 2014;27(2):141-6.

[11] Appiah-Dwomoh EK, Müller S, Mayer F. Is there an association between variables of static and dynamic postural control in adolescent athletes with back pain? German J Exer Sport Res 2019;49(2):150-5.

[12] Vassileva D, Nedelcheva I, Mindova S, Karaganova I. The Influence of Gait Pattern with AIDS on the patient's recovery in an early period of total knee replacement. Acta Med Bulgarica 2019;46(2):36-40.

[13] Mellalieu SD, Neil R, Hanton S, Fletcher D. Competition stress in sport performers: Stressors experienced in the competition environment. J Sports Sci 2009;27(7):729-44.

[14] Fullagar HH, Skorski S, Duffield R, Hammes D, Coutts AJ, Meyer T. Sleep and athletic performance: the effects of sleep loss on exercise performance, and physiological and cognitive responses to exercise. Sports Med 2015;45(2):161-86.

[15] Chang ECH, Chu CH, Karageorghis CI, Wang CC, Tsai JHC, Wang YS, et al. Relationship between mode of sport training and general cognitive performance. J Sport Health Sci 2017;6(1):89-95.

[16] Kross E, Berman MG, Mischel W, Walter Mischel, Edward E. Smith, Tor D, et al. Social rejection shares somatosensory representations with physical pain. Proc Natl Acad Sci 2011;108(15):6270-5.

[17] Han JH, Kim MJ, Yang HJ, Yu-Jin Lee, Yun-Hee Sung. Effects of therapeutic massage on gait and pain after delayed onset muscle soreness. J Exerc Rehabil 2014;10(2):136-40.

In: Pain Management ISBN: 978-1-68507-493-7
Editors: J Merrick and M Morad

Chapter 21

USING BDSM (BONDAGE/DISCIPLINE, DOMINANCE/SUBMISSION, SADISM/MASOCHISM) TO MANAGE ENDOMETRIOSIS PAIN

Kristina S Brown**, PhD, LMFT,
Leisel Iverson, MS, ATC and "Cari"
Couple and Family Therapy Department, Adler University, Chicago, Illinois and Psychology Department, Adler University, Chicago, Illinois, United States of America

ABSTRACT

Pain is the primary complaint of endometriosis sufferers to medical and behavioral health professionals. Management of pain for both functionality and improved quality of life varies across patient experiences. "Cari" is a 45-year-old woman who was first diagnosed with

* ***Correspondence:*** Kristina S Brown, PhD, LMFT, Couple and Family Therapy Department, Adler University, 17 N Dearborn, Chicago, IL 60602, United States. Email: kbrown@adler.edu.

endometriosis at the age of 23 years after already experiencing years of debilitating pain. Cari described her own journey as co-author of this case report including various methods of physician prescribed and illicit pain management including a history of self-harm. After years of suffering, Cari discovers BDSM (bondage/discipline, dominance/submission, sadism/masochism) which provides her with both relief from pain and improved quality of life. This case report emphasizes the need for broadening opportunities for utilizing alternative pain management of endometriosis and other pelvic pain disorders that are specific to each patient's needs.

INTRODUCTION

Endometriosis plagues one in ten ova-having individuals, e.g., biologically born women including non-binary and trans female persons. 72-87% of endometriosis cases present with chronic pelvic pain (CPP) as the main symptom (1). Both dysmenorrhea and dyspareunia impact the patient's quality of life including their primary and familial relationships and responsibilities across their personal and professional identities. Pain management is often a primary presenting goal that patients bring to medical and behavioral health specialists; "feeling pain is the main reason that people seek medical assistance" (2).

Behavioral health clinicians have long understood the use of self-harm as a method of managing emotional pain (3). For many, BDSM (bondage/discipline, dominance/submission, sadism/masochism) is considered a form of self-harm but the DSM5 de-pathologized it between consenting adults (4). Despite this, persons engaged in BDSM "have long been seen by medicine, the law, and caring professions as at best damaged (in need of therapy) and at worst (in need of legal or social regulation)" (5). For the patient, "Cari," presented in this case report, BDSM has become her primary intervention in the management of endometriosis pain subsequently improving her overall quality of life. This case study presentation is essential to help combat stigma regarding BDSM as a lifestyle across health care providers (6) as well as contribute to the literature on alternative interventions for endometriosis pain.

CASE REPORT

This case report focuses on the experiences of a 45-year-old biological woman diagnosed with endometriosis at the age of 23 years. The authors include direct quotes from the patient, "Cari," to provide the reader rich description of her illness narrative including discovering the benefits of BDSM to manage her endometriosis pain and improve her overall quality of life. Cari's own words are included in *italics* as a co-author of the report. Cari started menstruating at 11 years of age. By 13 years, she was *bleeding heavily every month for at least four, and often six days which required sanitary pads changes at least eight, and frequently 12 times, per day. The bleeding made me tired or exhausted and the pain made me restless, short-tempered, short-fused and angry.* Cari's clinical presentation of endometriosis includes a history of pain – both dysmenorrhea and dyspareunia.

At the age of 22 years, Cari collapsed on a cross-country flight. An onboard passenger who was a physician speculated that her appendix had ruptured and recommended the plane land immediately. An ER admission, several hours of medical testing and repeated physical examinations, revealed "no significant findings" despite unrelenting pain. Once Cari returned home, she learned that multiple ovarian cysts had simultaneously ruptured. Six months later, at the age of 23 years, Cari had her first laparoscopy and hysteroscopy and *a general surgeon scrubbed in to do an appendectomy because my OB/GYN said, "Given your recent history, the fewer potentially explosive organs down there, the better." That surgery was the official beginning of my endometriosis nightmare.*

Over the last 23 years, Cari has "collected" the following through her endometriosis pain management experience: a variety of cyclical and continuous birth control pills; eight laparoscopies (the eighth was via the da Vinci Surgical System), six with hysteroscopies and a presacral neurectomy accompanying the fifth laparoscopy and a cystoscopy with the seventh laparoscopy; three separate 6-month courses of Lupron Depot injections; a series of three cauda equina steroid injections spaced out across six months; six months of weekly pelvic floor dysfunction physical therapy; nine months of weekly acupuncturist needle insertion therapy with electric stimulation and burning moxa; a Mirena IUD; and a period of specific pain management treatment including a pain medication patch and weekly appointments with a psychologist.

In addition to surgeries and prescribed methods of pain management, Cari struggled with excesses of drugs and alcohol as self-medication for pain. *I was given prescription after prescription of opioids until I was taking five different opioids daily to manage the chronic pain caused by the endometriosis. Most days, it hurt to sit, stand, walk, drive, work out at the gym, and lay down in any position to sleep, and on really bad days, it hurt to take a deep breath. I continued to do what I had to do because staying still hurt even more. After months of failure by the opioids to even dull the edge of the increasing pain, I began mixing hard liquor and opioids out of desperation.* Cari described self-created regiments of hourly opioids with alcohol chasers throughout the evening just to sleep. At the age of 28 years, Cari was diagnosed with chronic pain-induced depression by the pain management psychologist and began a low dose of Prozac.

Cari also has a history of engaging in self-harming behaviors beginning as early as the age of seven years, when she would push straight pins through the skin of her fingertips. Adolescence included using hot liquid wax, matchbooks, and shaving. *I often turned the razor sideways to create long cuts on my thighs, Achilles tendon, or the area around my ankle bones. Running water over the fresh cuts made the pain electric and almost living as it scorched up my nerves to my brain.* In her 20s, Cari began her strength and conditioning coach career where she developed intensive exercise habits tuned to her own physical well-being. *Violating everything I believed and worked hard to teach, I pushed myself in the gym to the point of tearing soft tissue or breaking bone. Once I sustained an injury, I continued to work out. I partially ruptured my Achilles tendons five times, broke small bones in both feet/ankles and hands/wrists, strained muscles in my back, and tore ligaments or muscles in both my forearms, upper arms, and thighs. I rarely took anything for pain as I already knew it did little to nothing to manage my endometriosis pain. I pushed through the pain, knowing it was nothing compared to what lived deep inside my pelvis and abdomen.*

At the age of 38 years, Cari met her husband and learned about BDSM and *my life changed for the better forever. As our friendship grew into love, he became my dominant and I became his submissive. I accepted his collar and became his submissive months before he proposed, and we became engaged. Our marriage was as much an affirmation of marriage vows as our relationship as dominant and submissive. A curious thing happened during and after scenes. For the first time in my life, I was truly endometriosis pain-free for hours or days, depending on the intensity of the scene. The sex was amazing, but more than the sex it was the overwhelming stimulation and endorphin rush I experienced from the intense sensory overload provided by the ever-changing scenes involving different variations of spanking, flogging, paddling, breath play, blindfold usage, and other sensory deprivations or enhancements. It took me a while to recognize what was happening, but once I did, I began to crave our scenes for the calm and stillness I felt in my body following play.* Cari described an overall improvement of quality of life as her experiences of endometriosis pain decreased in response to regular sessions of BDSM.

DISCUSSION

Women like Cari with a long history of endometriosis are no stranger to pain. Often, they share narrative histories of different conventional, unconventional, and sometimes harmful attempts at endometriosis pain management. Cari shared all the different ways she tried to manage her pain, some which provided short-term relief, and other alternatives that were illicit and harmful, but by her report, nothing as impactful and effective as BDSM.

Success around pain management for endometriosis has been demonstrated through surgical intervention, medication including NSAIDs and GnRH antagonists, and hormonal therapies. Despite this, there are relapses of debilitating pain that plague both physicians/clinicians and patients, even after a hysterectomy (7). Infertility is a symptom and consequence of endometriosis with its' own experiences of mental and emotional pain. Dysmenorrhea and dyspareunia as well as other pain experiences due to endometriosis have serious implications for a woman's overall quality of life and mental health. Facchin et al. (8) confirmed the importance of exploring pain management and the inclusion of psychological intervention finding that "only pelvic pain had a negative impact on all the dependent variables and was associated with lower quality of life and higher anxiety and depression" (8). With the lack of generalizable success in the field of medicine, a broader exploration of nonmedical interventions is necessary.

Research on complementary and alternative treatments such as pelvic floor therapy, spinal cord stimulation (9), mindfulness (10), music therapy (11), yoga (12), acupuncture (13), Ayurvedic treatment (14) and thermal biofeedback (15) provides endometriosis sufferers with options to manage the pain they experience. Patients select interventions that both fit their lifestyle and are effective in their pain management. This case report adds to the literature with the goal of further broadening alternative pain management options sensitive to distinctive patient needs. Additionally, incorporating BDSM into a pain treatment plan not only for endometriosis, but for other pelvic pain experiences encourages acceptance across relevant treating medical professions of kink-oriented lifestyles.

Erotogenic masochism

The American psychologist Richard Solomon (1918-1995) (16) expanded the 1878 opponent process theory model developed by Ewald Hering (1834-1918), a German physiologist. This theory explains the connection between pain and pleasure that is seemingly antithetical. This theory can be utilized to further understand why patients self-harm. Pain, whether emotional or physical, can blindside a person. By taking charge of the pain experience through BDSM, the individual gains control of their physical pain experience by drawing pleasure. Pain is often experienced as a loss of control. In BDSM, the start and stop, persons involved, implements used, and scene location and duration are discussed before the session begins which return pleasure and pain control to the individuals involved in BDSM. Regaining control, even if only partial and temporary, quiets the constant roar of pain from, e.g., endometriosis, so the individual can reconnect with the self in ways blocked or forgotten by overstimulated physiological and psychological systems that are hyper-distressed.

CONCLUSION

This case report serves to educate the field on an alternative intervention that may meet the needs of some endometriosis patients and others experiencing chronic pelvic pain. The presented case of Cari includes a growing level of hyposensitivity to pain including a long history of pain and self-harm that intersects with a well-documented history of endometriosis. Cari experienced escalating pain that was inadequately managed by medical and accepted complementary and alternative treatments and interventions as well as illicit and detrimental measures. The presented case demonstrates how Cari explored her lifestyle choices and discovered an unconventional and nontraditional pain management approach which provided her a renewed sense of control, agency, and hope.

ACKNOWLEDGMENTS

There was no funding for this case report. The authors declare that they have no conflict of interest. Informed consent was obtained from "Cari" as co-author of this case report. The uniqueness of this case report is that it includes first person contributions from the patient, Cari, who prefers to stay anonymous. Her willingness to share her endometriosis story as a co-author allows us to provide an authentic voice for the readers of this case report. This study was conducted in accordance with the 1964 Declaration of Helsinki and its subsequent amendments.

References

[1] Muraleedharan A, Unnikrishnan P, Narayan P, Bhatt HSK. Ayurdevic treatment protocol for chronic pelvic pain in endometriosis. J Clin Diagnostic Res 2018;12(12):1-3.

[2] Leknes S, Bastian B. The benefits of pain. Rev Philosophy Psychol 2014;5:57-70.

[3] Brown TB, Kimball T. Cutting to live: A phenomenology of self-harm. J Marital Fam Ther 2013;39(2):195-208.

[4] Simula BL. Pleasure, power, and pain: A review of the literature on the experiences of BDSM participants. Sociol Compass 2018;13:1-24.

[5] Richters J, de Visser RO, Rissel CE, Grulich AE,d Smith AMA. Demographic and psychosocial features of participants in bondage and discipline, "sadomasochism" or dominance and submission (BDSM): Data from a national survey. J Sex Med 2008;5:1660-8.

[6] Waldura JF, Arora I, Randall AM, Farala JP, Sprott RA. Fifty shades of stigma: Exploring the health care experiences of kink-oriented patients. J Sex Med 2016;13:1918-29.

[7] Badiu CD, Sima MR, Mehedintu C, Mastalier B, Mandu M. Abdominial-pelvic pain in female patients with endometriosis – a review of the literature. Jf Mind Med Sci 2018;5(2):158-62.

[8] Facchin F, Barbara G, Saita E, Erzegovesi S, Martoni R, Vercellini R. Personality in women with endometriosis: Temperament and character dimensions and pelvic pain. Hum Reprod 2014;31(7):1515-21.

[9] Kapural L, Narouze SN, Janicki TI, Mekhail N. Spinal cord stimulation is an effective treatment for the chronic intractable visceral pelvic pain. Pain Med 2006;7(5):440-3.

[10] Kold M, Hansen T, Vedsted-Hansen H, Forman A. Mindfulness-based psychological intervention for coping with pain in endometriosis. Nord Psychol 2012;64(1):2-16.

[11] Colwell CM. Music as distraction and relaxation to reduce chronic pain and narcotic ingestion: A case study. Music Ther Perspect 1997;15(1):24-31.

[12] Gonçalves AV, Makuch MY, Setubal MS, Barros NF, Bahamondes L. A qualitative study on the practice of yoga for women with pain-associated endometriosis. J Altern Complement Med 2016;22(12):977-82.

[13] Mira TAA, Buen MM, Borges MG, Yela DA, Benetti-Pinto CL. Systematic review and meta-analysis of complementary treatments for women with symptomatic endometriosis. Int J Gynecol Obstet 2018;143: 2-9.

[14] Hawkins RS, Hart AD. The use of thermal biofeedback in the treatment of pain associated with endometriosis: Preliminary findings. Appl Psychophysiol Biofeedback 2003;28(4):279-89.

[15] Solomon R. The opponent-process theory of acquired motivation: The costs of pleasure and the benefits of pain. Am Psychologist 2008;35(8): 691-712.

SECTION FOUR: ACKNOWLEDGEMENTS

In: Pain Management
Editors: J Merrick and M Morad
ISBN: 978-1-68507-493-7

ABOUT THE EDITORS

Joav Merrick, MD, MMedSci, DMSc, born and educated in Denmark is professor of pediatrics, Division of Pediatrics, Hadassah Hebrew University Medical Center, Mt Scopus Campus, Jerusalem, Israel and Kentucky Children's Hospital, University of Kentucky, Lexington, Kentucky United States and professor of public health at the Center for Healthy Development, School of Public Health, Georgia State University, Atlanta, United States, the former medical director of the Health Services, Division for Intellectual and Developmental Disabilities, Ministry of Social Affairs and Social Services, Jerusalem, the founder and director of the National Institute of Child Health and Human Development in Israel. Numerous publications in the field of pediatrics, child health and human development, rehabilitation, intellectual disability, disability, health, welfare, abuse, advocacy, quality of life and prevention. Received the Peter Sabroe Child Award for outstanding work on behalf of Danish Children in 1985 and the International LEGO-Prize ("The Children's Nobel Prize") for an extraordinary contribution towards improvement in child welfare and well-being in 1987. In 2017 appointed a Kentucky Colonel by the Commonwealth of Kentucky, the highest honor the governor can bestow to a person. Email: jmerrick@zahav.net.il.

Mohammed Morad, MD, FRCP, born in Israel and educated in the Czech Republic, Israel and the United Kingdom. Professor of Pediatrics at

Kentucky Children's Hospital, University of Kentucky, Lexington, Kentucky, United States and Senior Lecturer at the Family Medicine Department, Community Health Division, Ben Gurion University of the Negev, Beer Sheva, Israel. Director of Yaski Teaching Medical Center, affiliated with Ben Gurion University in the Negev. Head of the Patient Safety Circle, Israel Federation of Family Physicians and Member of the Chamber of Ethics in Israel. Member of the Society of Patient Safety and Risk Management, Life Style Medicine, Pain Management and Rural Health Circle under the Israel Federation of Family Physicians. Lecturer on patient safety at Ben Gurion and Tel Aviv University. Researcher and publications in disability studies, Bedouin health research and patient safety. Received the Medical Director Award 2006 from the medical director of the Ministry of Social Affairs, Jerusalem. FRCP of the Royal College of Phyisicians in Edinburgh and the Royal College of Physicians and Surgeons in Glasgow, United Kingdom. Email: morad62@gmail.com.

In: Pain Management
Editors: J Merrick and M Morad
ISBN: 978-1-68507-493-7

About the National Institute of Child Health and Human Development in Israel

The National Institute of Child Health and Human Development (NICHD) in Israel was established in 1998 as a virtual institute under the auspices of the Medical Director, Ministry of Social Affairs and Social Services in order to function as the research arm for the Office of the Medical Director. In 1998 the National Council for Child Health and Pediatrics, Ministry of Health and in 1999 the Director General and Deputy Director General of the Ministry of Health endorsed the establishment of the NICHD.

Mission

The mission of a National Institute for Child Health and Human Development in Israel is to provide an academic focal point for the scholarly interdisciplinary study of child life, health, public health, welfare, disability, rehabilitation, intellectual disability and related aspects of human development. This mission includes research, teaching, clinical work, information and public service activities in the field of child health and human development.

Service and academic activities

Over the years many activities became focused in the south of Israel due to collaboration with various professionals at the Faculty of Health Sciences (FOHS) at the Ben Gurion University of the Negev (BGU). Since 2000 an affiliation with the Zusman Child Development Center at the Pediatric Division of Soroka University Medical Center has resulted in collaboration around the establishment of the Down Syndrome Clinic at that center. In 2002 a full course on "Disability" was established at the Recanati School for Allied Professions in the Community, FOHS, BGU and in 2005 collaboration was started with the Primary Care Unit of the faculty and disability became part of the master of public health course on "Children and society". In the academic year 2005-2006 a one semester course on "Aging with disability" was started as part of the master of science program in gerontology in our collaboration with the Center for Multidisciplinary Research in Aging. In 2010 collaborations with the Division of Pediatrics, Hadassah Hebrew University Medical Center, Jerusalem, Israel around the National Down Syndrome Center and teaching students and residents about intellectual and developmental disabilities as part of their training at this campus.

Research activities

The affiliated staff have over the years published work from projects and research activities in this national and international collaboration. In the year 2000 the International Journal of Adolescent Medicine and Health and in 2005 the International Journal on Disability and Human Development of De Gruyter Publishing House (Berlin and New York) were affiliated with the National Institute of Child Health and Human Development. From 2008 also the International Journal of Child Health and Human Development (Nova Science, New York), the International Journal of Child and Adolescent Health (Nova Science) and the Journal of Pain Management (Nova Science) affiliated and from 2009 the International

Public Health Journal (Nova Science) and Journal of Alternative Medicine Research (Nova Science). All peer-reviewed international journals.

National collaborations

Nationally the NICHD works in collaboration with the Faculty of Health Sciences, Ben Gurion University of the Negev; Department of Physical Therapy, Sackler School of Medicine, Tel Aviv University; Autism Center, Assaf HaRofeh Medical Center; National Rett and PKU Centers at Chaim Sheba Medical Center, Tel HaShomer; Department of Physiotherapy, Haifa University; Department of Education, Bar Ilan University, Ramat Gan, Faculty of Social Sciences and Health Sciences; College of Judea and Samaria in Ariel and in 2011 affiliation with Center for Pediatric Chronic Diseases and National Center for Down Syndrome, Department of Pediatrics, Hadassah Hebrew University Medical Center, Mount Scopus Campus, Jerusalem.

International collaborations

Internationally with the Department of Disability and Human Development, College of Applied Health Sciences, University of Illinois at Chicago; Strong Center for Developmental Disabilities, Golisano Children's Hospital at Strong, University of Rochester School of Medicine and Dentistry, New York; Centre on Intellectual Disabilities, University of Albany, New York; Centre for Chronic Disease Prevention and Control, Health Canada, Ottawa; Chandler Medical Center and Children's Hospital, Kentucky Children's Hospital, Section of Adolescent Medicine, University of Kentucky, Lexington; Chronic Disease Prevention and Control Research Center, Baylor College of Medicine, Houston, Texas; Division of Neuroscience, Department of Psychiatry, Columbia University, New York; Institute for the Study of Disadvantage and Disability, Atlanta; Center for Autism and Related Disorders, Department

Psychiatry, Children's Hospital Boston, Boston; Department of Pediatric and Adolescent Medicine, Western Michigan University Homer Stryker MD School of Medicine, Kalamazoo, Michigan, United States; Department of Paediatrics, Child Health and Adolescent Medicine, Children's Hospital at Westmead, Westmead, Australia; International Centre for the Study of Occupational and Mental Health, Düsseldorf, Germany; Centre for Advanced Studies in Nursing, Department of General Practice and Primary Care, University of Aberdeen, Aberdeen, United Kingdom; Quality of Life Research Center, Copenhagen, Denmark; Nordic School of Public Health, Gottenburg, Sweden, Scandinavian Institute of Quality of Working Life, Oslo, Norway; The Department of Applied Social Sciences (APSS) of The Hong Kong Polytechnic University Hong Kong.

Targets

Our focus is on research, international collaborations, clinical work, teaching and policy in health, disability and human development and to establish the NICHD as a permanent institute in Israel in order to conduct model research and policy.

Contact

Professor Joav Merrick, MD, MMedSci, DMSc
Director, National Institute of Child Health and Human Development, Jerusalem, Israel.
E-mail: jmerrick@zahav.net.il

SECTION FIVE: INDEX

INDEX

A

B

C

D

E

F

G

H

I

J

K

L

M

N